The Doctor's Kitchen

Dr Rupy Aujla

Supercharge
your Health with
100 Delicious
Everyday
Recipes

HarperCollins

To my mother. Without her love and guidance I would not be the doctor I am today … or a cook. I owe her everything.

HarperCollinsPublishers
1 London Bridge Street
London SE1 9GF

www.harpercollins.co.uk

First published by HarperCollinsPublishers 2017

10 11 12 13 14 15

A catalogue record of this book is available from the British Library

Photographer: Faith Mason
Food Stylist: Marina Filippelli
Prop Stylist: Sarah Birks
Senior Project Editor: Georgina Atsiaris

ISBN 978-0-00-823933-6

Printed and bound by GPS Group

MIX
Paper from responsible sources
FSC™ C007454

This book is produced from independently certified FSC™ paper to ensure responsible forest management.

For more information visit: www.harpercollins.co.uk/green

@doctors_kitchen

@doctors_kitchen

@thedoctorskitchen

www.thedoctorskitchen.com

The Doctor's Kitchen

Dr Rupy Aujla

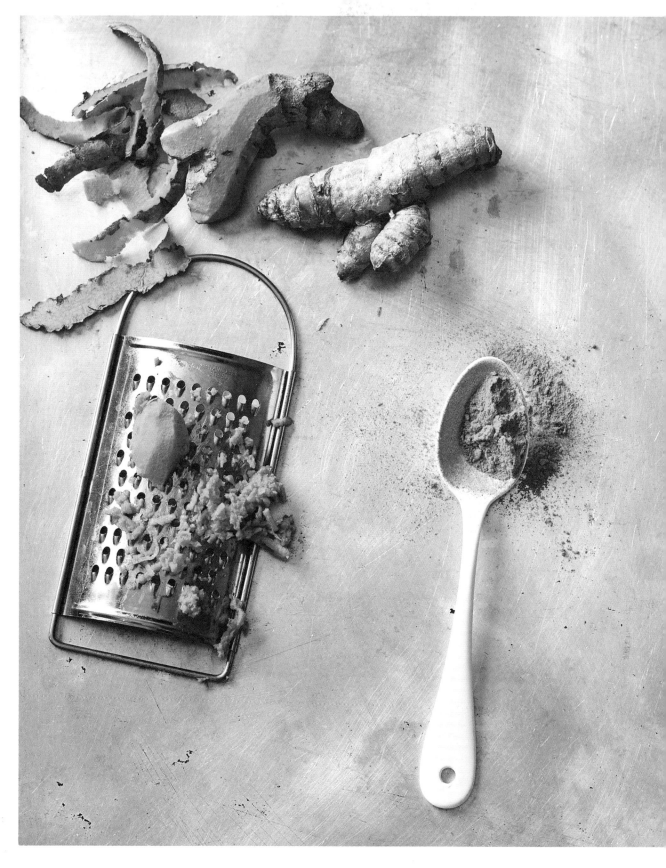

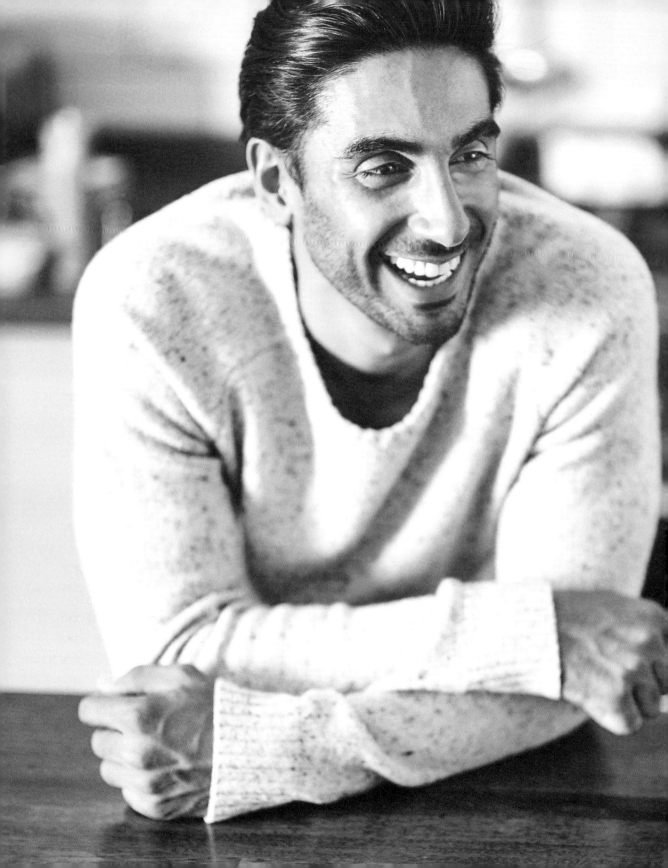

Introduction: Food as Medicine

Hi, I'm Rupy. I love practising medicine as a doctor in the NHS and I also have a real passion for showing my patients and colleagues the health benefits of food.

I believe what you choose to put on your plate is the most important health intervention anyone can make.

Imagine a world where everybody appreciates the true impact of diet and lifestyle on disease and is empowered to make permanent, simple changes. Some of the most prevalent illnesses can be alleviated and managed by making educated modifications to what we eat and how we live. We have been conditioned to believe that the sole purpose of going to the doctor is to get prescriptions and pills to cure us when we are sick, but my aspiration is to teach patients to take control of their health and prevent illness from occurring in the first place by using a lifestyle medicine approach.

Every day, we make choices that either positively or negatively impact our bodies. But I haven't written this book to scare you into a restrictive and bland way of life. I'm here to welcome you on a journey of colour, flavour and cultures that makes healthy eating delicious and accessible to everyone. I want to introduce you to the medicinal effects of food, while showing you how it can be vibrant and easy to slot into a hectic lifestyle.

As a GP in the NHS, I see hundreds of patients every week. From my desk I witness the outcome of poor diet and lifestyle time and time again: high blood pressure, low mood, chronic pain, diabetes, cognitive decline. The reality is, we are not taught the immense value of nutrition in our communities, or even as students at medical school. Addressing this problem will combat some of the most common and preventable illnesses in society.

I'm still practising as a doctor, so I understand that a busy working life and a lack of cooking skills have an impact on what we choose to eat. If we learn about the importance of food, we can stop it from slipping down our list of priorities. I'm here to help you navigate those roadblocks and motivate you to experiment with ingredients that have amazing benefits. You'll discover the health qualities of everyday ingredients and discover the tools to cook delicious meals all the time.

After spending 15 years training in medicine, learning about human biochemistry and the effects of disease, my attention is now focused on the study of nutrition, the impact of food on our genes, our brain and our gut, and the power of a healthy lifestyle. As well as explaining the science, I aim to educate and inspire you to want to cook.

The foundation for your health journey starts on your plate and it's more powerful than any pill I can prescribe.

You'll realise why I believe a good understanding of nutrition is essential for everybody, at all stages of life. The foundation for your health journey starts on your plate and it's more powerful than any pill I can prescribe.

Nature has some incredible foods that ancient cultures have appreciated for thousands of years. Furthermore, the use of spices and herbs adds a wealth of aroma, warmth and enjoyment to cooking, and the intricate

chemistry of these ingredients has a profound effect on our bodies. I hope to persuade you that adding these types of foods to your diet is fundamental to feeling energetic and youthful long into your life.

I'm here to smash the preconception that a healthy way of life is expensive and shed the pretence that any single book can be a 'one-stop shop' to changing your entire life. Today is simply the starting point. I will guide you through living-well principles so that you can create a plan of change yourself (if you need one at all) that suits your needs, motivation and lifestyle. Everyone stands to benefit from the recipes and tips in this book.

This is my unbiased, current and evidence-based medical opinion on healthy eating. Today's 'wellness' industry can lack scientific credibility and has occasionally spread misinformation that is harmful to your health. The overwhelming, conflicting messages can be difficult to navigate, especially to those who are just starting out. It's time we moved away from cherry-picking strands of evidence to support faddy diets and finally provide everyone with the wealth of knowledge available. Using science and my clinical perspective as guiding principles, this book gives you the delicious recipes and life tools that you need to feel fantastic and stay well.

You don't need to know the fancy chemistry, the correct proportions of 'macros' or how to use calorie counters and scales. The majority of us just need to stick to sound diet and lifestyle principles (that I'll introduce you to in this book), and our health will flourish.

Expect to feel happier with your weight, calmer in your mind and, overall, more content knowing that the changes you make are sustainable for life. The ability to reverse disease, improve mental health and feel fantastic has never tasted so good.

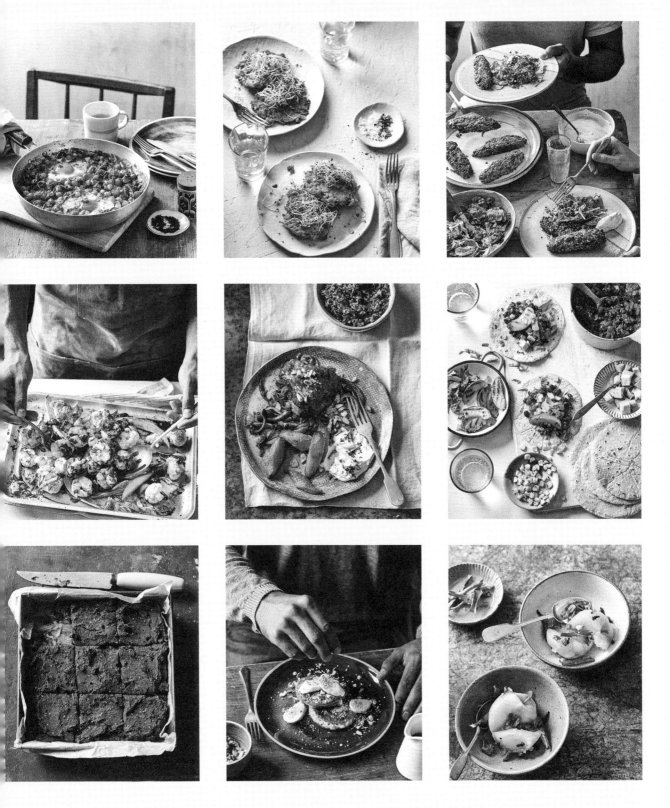

Introduction

Food and medicine go hand in hand and sometimes changing our diet can be the best intervention.

At the age of 12, I witnessed my mother take control of her medical condition that had baffled multiple physicians. She used to suffer random anaphylaxis attacks; the worst form of allergy where your airway can close and your blood pressure drops. The attacks are life threatening and require treatment with an adrenaline shot. After undergoing a barrage of medical tests to find a cause, none was found. As a last resort, her doctors recommended lifelong allergy medications, which unfortunately have a range of side effects. These included crushing fatigue and intolerable nausea but, worst of all, they didn't completely eradicate the attacks. The daily unease of potentially having an episode was incredibly stressful for her.

Not content with being reliant on drugs that weren't completely working, she decided to make radical changes to her daily life. Her Indian upbringing had instilled in her the value of food. As a trained lawyer, she used her research skills and analytical approach to examine the scientific literature and create a plan of action. I watched her completely overhaul her diet and lifestyle, while simultaneously running her businesses, our household and raising two demanding children. Her daily 'prescription' included a wholefoods diet packed with vegetables, good sleep patterns, exercise and meditation. She became more confident, stronger and gradually came off all medications with the support of her doctors. Thankfully, she has never needed to use an adrenaline shot again. This was my earliest introduction to the power of 'food as medicine'.

My mother's experience drove me to want to be a doctor. I worked hard to earn myself a place at Imperial College London. I started medical school with the understanding and strong belief that food could be as powerful as pharmaceuticals. However, despite being intrigued by 'alternative therapies' at a young age, I wanted to immerse myself in conventional medical training. The body has always fascinated me. Learning the anatomy, biochemistry and foundations of how we function was an incredible experience, but noticeably lacking from the curricula was an emphasis on nutrition. What we put into our bodies on a daily basis is just as important as medication, but I wasn't taught to appreciate the power of lifestyle and food. Only when I became ill myself would I remember what inspired me to become a doctor in the first place.

After medical school, I experienced two gruelling years as a junior doctor in central London hospitals. The stress and responsibility on a newly trained medic is unfathomable. Within two weeks of qualifying, I found myself wandering the corridors of a hospital alone, at night, armed with nothing but a stethoscope and two bleeps, providing the sole junior cover for medical wards. No amount of book smart prepares you for hospital life.

I began to realise how self-sacrificing healthcare workers are for the service. We eat poorly, work awkward hours and the stress is

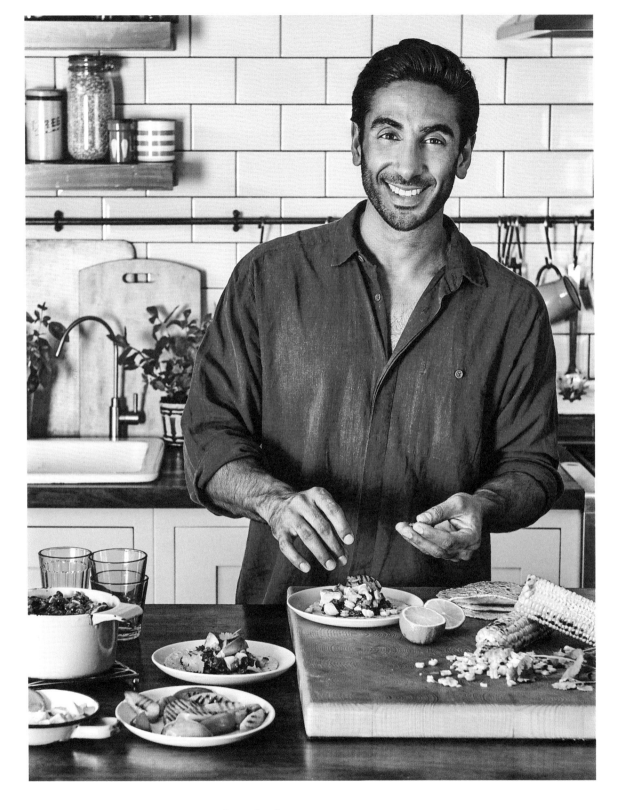

Introduction

intense. Our environment often dictates what we can eat, and in the interest of convenience, the choice is often a poor one. It's no wonder that on average our lives are shorter, we're more likely to suffer mental-health issues and obesity is greater among us than the general population. We are certainly not pillars of good health to look up to!

For the next year
I focused on my
lifestyle and replaced
elements in my diet,
all while juggling the
hectic job of being
a junior doctor.

I remember vividly, in the last few hours of my weekend shift (after working for 12 consecutive days), I noticed I was having palpitations. I asked my registrar to check my pulse and within the hour I was admitted to the acute medical unit. They found I was in fast atrial fibrillation (AF), a condition where your heart beats irregularly, inefficiently and, in my case, very fast. Up to 200 beats per minute. Luckily, I didn't require emergency treatment (a cardioversion, where an electronic shock is used to revert the heart rhythm back to a normal one), but this episode of atrial fibrillation was to be the first of many over the next two years.

I went on to suffer AF episodes weekly throughout my junior doctor training. I would often have to take medication to revert my heart rhythm, which had some unpleasant side effects. Despite these episodes I continued to work – nothing was going to stand in the way of me being a doctor. My condition was rare in someone of my age, so I was a very unusual case. I underwent multiple investigations to find a cause; stress tests, ECGs, cardiac MRIs, bloods, electrophysiology testing, echocardiograms, none of which revealed a reason for it. According to my doctors I was otherwise in 'great health'.

After discussing my case with some respected cardiologists, I was offered a choice of lifelong medication or a relatively new intervention called an ablation, a procedure where an area near the heart is 'burnt' using an accurate fine laser. It carries some serious potential complications including stroke, perforation to the heart and death. Despite the seriousness of the condition, I could control the episodes with high-dose drugs while I decided whether to opt for the ablation. With the blessing of my cardiologists, I followed in the footsteps of my mother and self-experimented with some alternatives while I weighed up the option of having a procedure.

For the next year I focused on my lifestyle and replaced elements in my diet, all while juggling the hectic job of being a junior doctor. I read everything I could on associations between diet and my condition, and entered a new world of wellness. Out went cereals and toast for breakfast, in came dark green leafy vegetables with miso, nuts and seeds. Gone were the soggy sandwiches at lunch: I never left for work without my Tupperware brimming with cruciferous vegetables cooked in delicious spices and tasty fats. I began to realise the impact of stress on my heart, so I started meditating. I appreciated the importance of sleep, so I made sure (when I wasn't on night shifts!) I was tucked up on time. More importantly, I never sacrificed my enjoyment for life. I wasn't to be owned or dictated to by a condition. I wanted to take control of it … if I could.

My AF episodes reduced from one or two a week to zero.

On discussing my experiences with cardiologists, general physicians and lifestyle medicine practitioners it was hard to retrospectively pinpoint exactly what had happened to make the AF episodes stop. My increased vegetable intake likely replaced electrolytes and vitamins in my cells that were lacking. Eating cruciferous vegetables on a daily basis flooded my body with plant chemicals that we now understand have profound effects on DNA. I continued to drink alcohol on occasion, but I removed sugary drinks completely. My added dietary fibre is likely to have improved the functioning of my gut bacteria, which can lower inflammation via a variety of chemical pathways.

I potentially attenuated the stress in my life triggered by poor sleep and a demanding job by increasing essential fatty acids in my food and practising mindfulness.

Rather than focusing on ridding myself of a condition, I had concentrated my efforts on providing my body with the best environment I could. I worked at being well in mind and body as much as possible. The complex interplay of food on our physiology, our DNA and even the microbes residing in our gut is a universe of science in itself. Without delving further into the analysis, what my experience reaffirmed for me was the immense power of lifestyle and the incredible ability of the body to 'self heal' if given the correct nutrition.

My family's story, my personal story and those of the thousands of patients across the world who have managed to reverse and prevent disease using lifestyle medicine is my motivation for writing this book. This is my opportunity to share the information I've gleaned on my journey so far, and the journey I am still on.

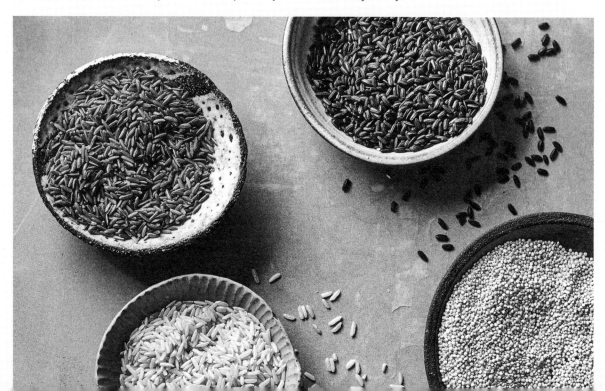

Medical experience

My GP training was brilliant. I was experienced in multiple medical specialities, equipped to diagnose and skilled at providing emotional support. However, I was horribly inept at addressing the root cause of the biggest problems facing primary care across the globe: lifestyle-related illness, including diabetes, obesity and heart disease.

Beyond the ineffective recommendations of a low-fat, low-calorie diet we propose for weight loss and cholesterol control, there are no tailored diets for conditions. From my personal experience, I knew there was much more to food than just a collection of macronutrients and the simplistic view that we eat for energy purposes. I was ill equipped to give advice because nutrition training at medical school was lacklustre. So, to help myself and my patients, I decided to do the research.

I scoured journals, watched presentations, attended international nutrition conferences and began to unravel a magnitude of clinical evidence highlighting the impact of food on disease. I read thousands of papers, studies, editorials and books dedicated to nutritional medicine, and was shocked that medical schools cover this entire body of evidence in just a few uninspiring lectures.

I began to start my consultations by enquiring what patients would eat on a daily basis: how do you start your day? What time do you eat at night? Do you snack incessantly after meals? My clinics were more engaging and my patients loved the emphasis on nutrition. Convincing them that the key to longevity and good health was accessible using delicious recipes that I would tailor to their lifestyle, was motivational. I was able to inspire people to take control of their conditions through food in a way I hadn't done before with just medications. I began to focus on promoting wellness habits, rather than just diagnosing disease.

My diabetic patients would improve their blood-sugar control, arthritic patients would lose weight and become more active and even those who had no significant change in their body composition felt better in themselves. Realising that I could combine my passion for recipe creating and flavour with a career dedicated to healing people was a revelation for me.

But, I couldn't keep writing recipes for every patient in my consulting room. I was seeing over 40 patients a day, plus home visits, plus paperwork and prescriptions. It was just not sustainable. And that's when the idea of 'The Doctor's Kitchen' was born: a multi-platform resource inspiring patients to appreciate the beauty of food and the medicinal effects of eating well. A YouTube channel, Instagram account and blog where I could confidently direct patients to gain evidence-based information, lend my perspective on healthy eating and teach them how to cook their way to health.

An accumulation of poor dietary and lifestyle choices often leads patients to the emergency room and it's partly my experience in A&E that's brought me on this journey. It's often a surprise to patients when their emergency doctor starts enquiring about their dietary habits, but acute care and chronic disease are related in many ways. Sometimes it's a culmination of factors that results in tragedies like a heart attack, stroke or even a nasty skin infection that's linked to poor diabetes control. Separating diet and lifestyle from acute medicine blinds us to the solution for our overburdened healthcare systems. I truly believe the answer lies in the quality of our community care where food plays a pivotal role. Practising good nutrition and lifestyle medicine means we can pre-empt disease rather than react to it in the emergency department.

Plates over pills

I want to make this clear so there is no doubt on this statement: food is medicine. It's not my opinion, I'm not saying it because it's fashionable and trendy, it's quite frankly a fact.

We have a library of studies that demonstrate the effectiveness of nutritional interventions on lifestyle diseases that are society's biggest killers. My job is to give you a flavour of the science and encourage you to value the importance of mealtimes. We need to understand that what we put into our bodies dictates how they function and deal with illness.

When I refer to food as 'medicine' I'm not talking about simply using 'natural medications' or food supplements instead of pharmaceuticals. I don't advocate swapping your cholesterol-lowering drugs for a bag of nuts if you have abnormal biochemistry, for example. A traditional pharmaceutical model of healthcare where symptoms are treated individually is not the answer to our Western healthcare woes. It's important that we don't look at food like a 'pill'. No magic bullet in the form of turmeric supplements, green tea shots or pomegranate juice exists, I'm afraid.

A complex interplay of diet, sleep, exercise and stress underlies the root cause of disease. This relationship between our environment and human biochemistry is alien to most conventionally trained doctors like myself, and we must redress the balance.[1] The reason why I'm so nutrition focused and I believe in the power of 'plates over pills' is because it's the easiest, most cost-effective and evidence-based method of

preventing and reversing disease. The effect of a Mediterranean diet on cancer,[2] diabetes[3] and cardiovascular risk[4,5] is a simple example of this statement in action. By improving patients' diets we can drastically reduce the likelihood of all three common debilitating conditions to a far greater degree than any number of pills or surgical interventions.[2,5]

This is the direction in which medicine should be heading. Nutrition, along with other lifestyle factors, is where we need to concentrate our studies and resources. I've come across enough research and had enough personal experience in clinic with patients to judge that nutritional medicine is not a fringe concept. Dietary strategies are being trialled to reverse diabetes[6,7] and even address the tricky and controversial subject of dementia.[8] The added advantage of taking a nutritional approach to tackling disease is the beneficial upshot of eating well, compared to the many side effects associated with medications. I'm always plagued with guilt whenever a patient suffers an adverse side effect from medication, of which there are many examples, from swollen legs as a result of blood-pressure drugs to an increased risk of fractures related to antacid medications.[9]

In general practice there is a clear need for medications, but where a cost-effective, evidence-based alternative exists and has a plausible mechanism of action I would encourage us as a scientific community to investigate and embrace it. I urge physicians and patients to explore the multitude of other treatment methods before we succumb to medications for chronic conditions. This needs to happen. Healthcare systems across the Western world are crumbling under the weight of growing financial demands[10,11] and no matter how much we invest in novel therapeutics we must always start with simple diet and lifestyle measures. I am here to empower you.

Discovering the plethora of studies demonstrating how effective lifestyle interventions are was revolutionary to me. In fact, our current guidelines for some of the most common lifestyle-related diseases reflect this. The first step to tackling diabetes, hypertension and high cholesterol according to the National Institute for Health and Care Excellence is 'Lifestyle Change'.[12,13,14] Yet most doctors wouldn't know where to start when it comes to giving dietary advice and this poor ability to motivate our patients to embrace a healthy outlook is reflected by how over-medicated we are as a population. I'm convinced that our indulgence in pills over plates is a product of poor nutrition training in the medical curricula, which still stands at less than 20 hours of teaching during a five-year medical degree.[15,16] If medical students were encouraged to learn more about the impact of lifestyle, we'd have a much healthier nation.[17,18] Our lack of knowledge, short consultation times and patient demand for a quick fix creates a scenario where the easiest option is to provide pharmaceuticals. But, the first thing we should be asking before reaching for that prescription pad is, 'What are you eating?'

Our population is plagued by obesity, stress and cardiovascular disease, and the prevalence of these conditions is rising fast.[19] The answer to our epidemic of chronic disease is staring at us from the grocery aisles. I want to prevent the need for invasive devices, powerful prescription medications or painful procedures and offer

The answer to our epidemic of chronic disease is staring at us from the grocery aisles.

a delightful alternative: eating fresh produce, colourful plants and igniting a passion for flavour! Best of all, the creativity and pleasure of preparing and eating good food is attainable for everyone.

Rather than using this section to bombard you with myriad papers, details of trials and large studies to prove a point, I've speckled all the recipes with bite-sized chunks of information to give you a sense of this interesting research. I've also included amongst the recipes some further information on my favourite ingredients and their amazing health benefits (see pages 68–69). You might expect 'health food' to be bland and lacking variety, but I'm going to show you it's the exact opposite. Flavour as well as function is what I'm passionate about, and diversity of ingredients is essential. Our health depends on it.

Health is not a privilege

As a GP in the NHS, I'm passionate about accessible healthcare for everyone. I am fully aware that people's circumstances are different and there is a perception that using fresh produce and eating well is expensive and attainable only for the privileged. It doesn't have to be.

Well-branded supplements, yoga on top of luxury hotels and eye-wateringly expensive turmeric lattes … You'd be forgiven for thinking a 'healthy' life was akin to an exclusive, invite-only club. Most of my colleagues expect me to cynically dismiss this trend. After all, it's damaging to people's self-esteem, it promotes an unhealthy attitude towards body image and excludes those in society that are the most vulnerable. But, actually, I believe we need to think beyond a 'them' and 'us' attitude. Despite its many flaws and shortcomings, the wellness industry has done an unbelievable job of motivating a generation of millennials to drink green smoothies, include kale as a staple in their shopping baskets, and exercise. No number of doctor visits could create such impressive behavioural change!

Without the allure of healthy living promoted by aspirational figures, 'food in medicine' wouldn't have gained such attention in recent years. So, while doctors and health professionals can be damning of the industry, I'm grateful for the spotlight and want to know, where we can steer this trend in the future?

My aim is to make healthy eating inclusive and accessible to all. I personally witness a sense of elitism around eating well and many

of my patients associate health with wealth. I'm constantly challenged in the consulting room by patients who believe they don't have the time or money for a good diet. I see patients from all walks of life and let me share this with you: just because you are well off doesn't automatically make you healthy, even if you can afford expensive ingredients.

Forget all of your preconceptions of 'wellness'.

The most nutritionally dense foods are the least expensive on the shelf. These are the real 'superfoods' available in supermarkets, and that's why I focus on them. Once you understand the principles of eating well, health doesn't become a privilege. It's a choice no more expensive than the average household can afford.

I'm proud to work with a lottery-funded community kitchen, Made in Hackney, to dispel these myths. We inform people about where to get local organic produce, veg drop boxes and, ultimately, how to use wholesome ingredients in our daily life cheaply and efficiently. As the only doctor in the organisation, I lend a clinical perspective to the kitchen sessions. It's humbling to have the opportunity to explore people's experiences of food in medicine and break the cycle of 'can't cook, won't cook' attitudes.

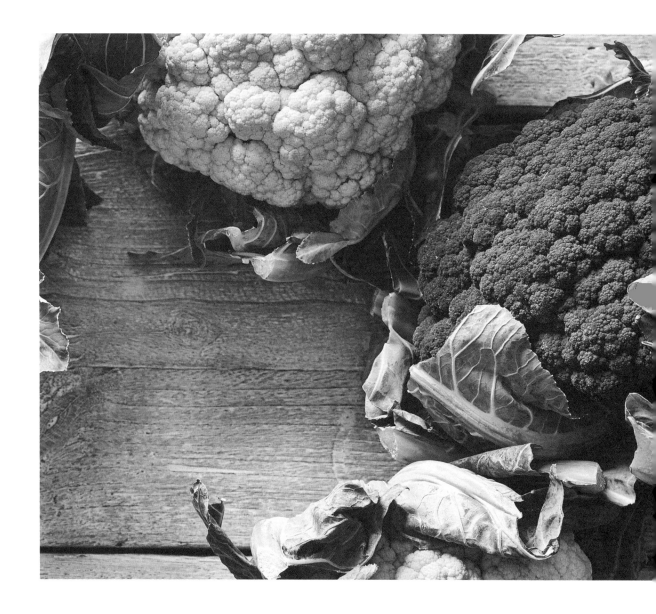

Think of the repercussions for public health if everybody nationwide had access to simple nutritional advice and was taught the fundamentals of healthy living? Healthy eating is attainable whatever your background. This isn't an exclusive club; it's how we shape the future of wellness.

The most nutritionally dense foods are the least expensive on the shelf.

Why I eat 'plant-focused'

On social media people often mistake me for a vegetarian or vegan because I get so excitable about vegetables. I do actually eat all types of meat and fish but I focus my diet around plants.

Rest assured there is logical reasoning underpinning my enthusiasm for chicory, cabbages and – of course – the greens! Abundant in vitamins and minerals, everybody generally knows they're 'good for us', but the story goes a lot deeper.

Phytochemicals, the chemicals found in plants, are another explanation for the incredible health benefits of fruits and vegetables.[20] These are what give plants their pigment, smell and, importantly, flavour.[21] It's the study of these chemicals that ignited my passion for nutritional medicine. A number of research papers look at their effect on inflammation,[22] bone health[23] and even cancer.[24] We have only scratched the surface when it comes to investigating just how influential these thousands of bioactive compounds are to human health. But, looking at the associations between food and disease, the positive impact of diets largely based on plants and whole foods is indisputable.[25] This is why they make up the bulk of my daily plate and why they should feature heavily on yours, too.

These compounds exist in a multitude of produce that is commonplace in grocery stores nationwide. Everything from a simple carrot to your basic apple is brimming with phytochemicals like quercetin and carotene.[26] These simple, affordable and accessible ingredients are key to good health. What's more, eating plates of a variety of colourful plants is the easiest way to guarantee a complete range of these phytochemicals,[27] which is why my dishes appear so vibrant. Using a multitude of herbs and spices (which have their own health benefits) to complement the ingredients is an easy undertaking for a home cook once you know how.

Having sifted through piles of studies involving thousands of people (followed up for years) and experiments examining the biological mechanisms behind the health-promoting effect of food, I can tell you the evidence is convincing. You can lower your risk of stroke, cancer and heart disease by increasing your fruit and vegetable intake.[28,25,29,30] Eat mostly plants and you'll stand a better chance at living a healthier, more vibrant and fulfilling life, free of disease.

I enjoy animal protein of all varieties – fish, poultry, chicken, game and beef – about once or twice a week. Animal products are an easy and delicious source of complete proteins. Key micronutrients such as zinc and vitamin B12 are nutritional qualities very hard to obtain in purely plant-based diets.[31] But, I see meat and animal products as a luxury item in the same way our ancestors would have treated them.[32,33]

On the subject of meat, I do have concerns about the harmful effects of cheaper mass-produced livestock on our health and the environment. On balance, a stressed, improperly reared animal is not likely to be good for us despite the benefits of convenient protein and nutrients. The type of feed, use of medications and the space an animal has been allowed to roam in all have an impact on their health and can negatively impact ours.[34]

The most well-studied diet we have access to has examined the eating habits of thousands of patients over decades. That is the Mediterranean diet. I am unapologetic for it not being a new, sexy, alternative eating plan that will grab headlines. Instead, it's solid, evidence-based nutritional advice about how the majority of us would benefit from eating.[35] It's a launch-pad to start a healthy lifestyle journey, I know it's safe and … it's actually quite vegetarian! It doesn't mean piles of pasta, bread and quick-releasing carbohydrates. It focuses on plant-based sources of protein and fibre, such as nuts and legumes, good-quality fat and a limit on meat intake.[36]

Eating based on the principles of a Mediterranean diet is a good starting point, and is one I personally follow. For these science-grounded arguments, I think focusing meals around plants is a good, well-established entry point for most people.

Instead of pushing a particular dietary dogma I want to encourage you to choose a fitter lifestyle by tempting your taste buds rather than making you eat vegetables because you feel you ought to. This way of eating doesn't have to be boring. I'm using the principles of this diet to create enticing multi-ethnic dishes that you can tweak according to your preferences. This journey is not limited in its culinary scope and I hope to show you why it's also medicinal.

Eat mostly plants and you'll stand a better chance at living a healthier, more vibrant and fulfilling life, free of disease.

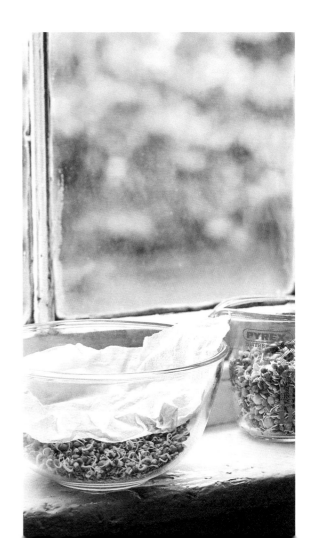

Introduction

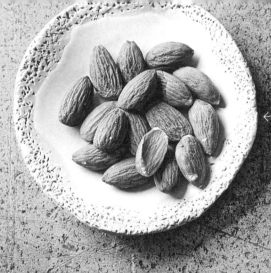

almonds

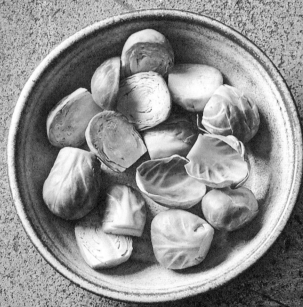

Brussel sprouts

sunflower seeds

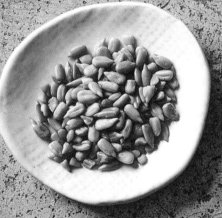

Nuts and seeds

Hemp seeds, cashews, peanuts, chia seeds, quinoa, almonds, Brazil nuts, pumpkin seeds, sunflower seeds

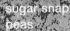

sugar snap peas

Greens

Broccoli, Brussel sprouts, asparagus, peas, sugar snap peas

hemp seeds

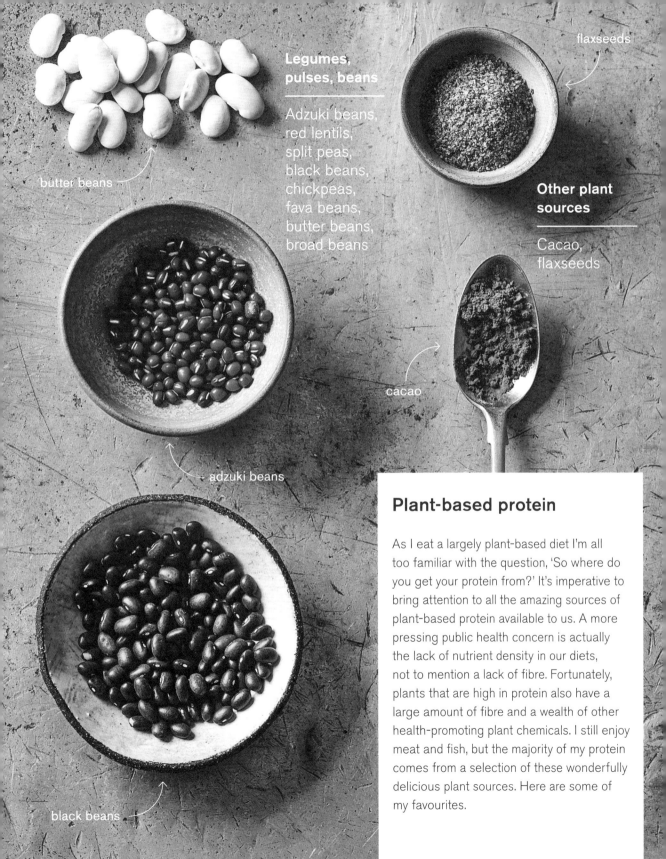

Legumes, pulses, beans

Adzuki beans, red lentils, split peas, black beans, chickpeas, fava beans, butter beans, broad beans

flaxseeds

Other plant sources

Cacao, flaxseeds

butter beans

cacao

adzuki beans

black beans

Plant-based protein

As I eat a largely plant-based diet I'm all too familiar with the question, 'So where do you get your protein from?' It's imperative to bring attention to all the amazing sources of plant-based protein available to us. A more pressing public health concern is actually the lack of nutrient density in our diets, not to mention a lack of fibre. Fortunately, plants that are high in protein also have a large amount of fibre and a wealth of other health-promoting plant chemicals. I still enjoy meat and fish, but the majority of my protein comes from a selection of these wonderfully delicious plant sources. Here are some of my favourites.

Health is in the gut of the beholder

I want to take you on a journey through recent scientific discoveries in nutrition that are shaping our knowledge of food in medicine. We could not start anywhere more exciting than with our digestive system.

Despite the exhausting and confusing gut-health messages in the media, the science behind our microbiome (the population of microbes that live in or around the body) is compelling. Studies looking at the microbiome have accelerated over the last decade and doctors are calling it 'the forgotten organ'.[37]

The trillions of microbes (including fungi, bacteria and viruses) largely concentrated in our colon are thought to protect us from infections,[38] break down molecules of food,[39] create neurotransmitters and even alter our immune system.[40,41] These microbes could impact diseases as far-ranging as dementia[42] and diabetes.[43] Neurologists, endocrinologists and psychiatrists are all looking at gut-focused treatments for a range of conditions we never thought were related. Even critical-care specialists who work in intensive care are getting involved in the conversation about how the gut impacts treatment of the sickest patients in hospital.[44]

The hype is real. Gut health is very important and the current discussion in medicine is going far beyond the expensive yoghurt drinks on supermarket shelves. Rather than a fad, I see the popularity of foods to help our microbiome as a return to traditional methods of eating that our ancestors developed. And there's evidence for this across all cultural backgrounds. In Japan, pickled ginger is consumed with sushi and miso broth is prepared before large meals. Indians drink

fermented yoghurt-based drinks ('lassi') and eat a range of pickles with curries. Middle Easterners enjoy kefir, Nordics have smörgåsgurka and Koreans love their kimchi. Spotting a trend? Fermented foods have a long, well-established history throughout different societies' eating habits, but a lot has changed in Western diets.

Food just doesn't have the same qualities it used to. We pasteurise, radiate and add a ton of additives to processed foods to make them sterile for convenience and shelf life. All of which have been shown to negatively impact the microbiome.[45]

This concept of bacteria being beneficial is alien to a lot of people because we're taught to think of them as harmful. But the vast majority of bacteria that live in our body are performing vital functions that allow us to maintain our health. These bacteria are in constant communication with our own cells and it's important we look after them. I want to encourage you to eat foods that protect and boost your microbiome while introducing bacteria back into your diet.

Eating a diet that nurtures our microbiome is what the current research lends itself toward, but that does not necessarily mean you need to consume expensive supplements and tinctures. Instead, here are some evidence-based and safe dietary interventions to improve your gut health ... deliciously!

• Prebiotic foods are where the power is! These are specialised types of fibre that are indigestible by the human intestine, but our microbes are able to break them down. Prebiotic fibres essentially feed our microbes and keep them healthy. Not only are they cheap and accessible, they bring a wealth of different flavours and textures to a meal. Jerusalem artichokes, asparagus stem, flax, chicory, wholegrains and pulses are great examples of fibre-rich foods your bugs and taste buds will love, and this book is full of examples of how to get them into your diet. I make everything from stews, meatballs and roasts from these ingredients. This 'health' food is delicious and easy to incorporate into your way of eating. Plus, by generally increasing all types of fibre, we can potentially reduce the incidence of cancers, cardiovascular disease and inflammation of the bowel.[46]

Eating a diet that nurtures our microbiome is what the current research lends itself toward, but that does not necessarily mean you need to consume expensive supplements and tinctures.

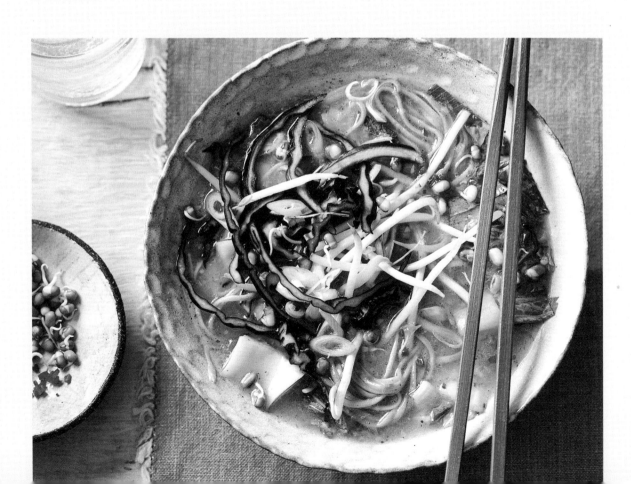

• Probiotic foods taste delicious and are a natural way of introducing live bacteria into your body. Despite the popularity of probiotic capsules and powders it's important to remember that none of these products is created equal. It's true that some research has shown benefits for urinary-tract disorders[47] and irritable bowel,[48] but the study of which bugs can potentially impact a condition is still very much in its infancy.[49,50]

For now, I encourage experimenting with different ingredients like traditionally prepared

I see the popularity of foods to help our microbiome as a return to traditional methods of eating …

kimchi, sauerkrauts and probiotic yoghurts that are full of different strains of bacteria that may have benefits.[51,52,53] Look for unpasteurised varieties usually found in the fridge section of supermarkets. Experiment by folding them through salads or simply adding them to the side of a dish as a garnish. They can complement the simplest of dishes and add another dimension of flavour.

• Polyphenol-rich foods like cacao, dark green leafy vegetables, beetroot and green tea are richly coloured and intensely flavoured ingredients that bring a host of benefits to your body.[54] Polyphenols are chemicals we find in plants of which there are literally thousands. Some of them have been shown to improve the gut lining, encourage growth of microbe patterns that are beneficial as well as have other advantages to general health. My recipes are designed to incorporate as many different polyphenol-rich foods as possible.

• Spice your food. Turmeric, cumin, sumac, cinnamon and caraway are just some of the ingredients that improve the aroma and taste of foods, but spices in general are another source of polyphenols. We'll talk more about them in the Medicinal Spices section (see page 43), but for now consider that the inclusion of these fabulous ingredients could potentially have positive effects on your gut bugs by reducing inflammation.[55]

• A varied diet is key. Your microbes thrive on new, interesting foods, which is why eating seasonally, for example, may encourage you to change things up throughout the year. We want to make sure your microbes are not bored with having the same meals and studies suggest they tend to favour diversity![56,57] There appears to be an improvement in the range of gut bacteria populations when a variety of foods are consumed, so here's yet another reason to try out some gorgeous, colourful recipes and mix things up.

• Raw foods. I'm not a raw foodist, nor do I advocate a completely raw diet. And, contrary to popular belief, cooking doesn't destroy all the micronutrients in foods. Sometimes, cooking can actually increase the availability of phytochemicals,[58] like in the case of tomatoes[59] and broccoli.[60] But, having some raw foods in your diet like celery, kohlrabi or radicchio is great for the bugs. It makes another argument for not overcooking your vegetables and keeping a little more texture to your food, too. Nobody likes overcooked sprouts!

When it comes to a holistic approach of how to look after our microbiomes there are some other suggestions outside of our diets that I encourage patients to think about as well.

• Avoid antibiotics. Your doctor is trained to recognise and prescribe these when there is a clear need for them, but far too often we see them used inappropriately.[61] Antibiotic medications indiscriminately remove large proportions of bacteria including the beneficial types that are good for us,[62] so I always encourage a reserved attitude to using and requesting them. You are more likely to convince your doctor to hand them over inappropriately by pressuring them, than if you trust their pragmatic and informed decision.

The Royal Colleges of medicine and editors of medical journals are very aware of the growing problem of antibiotic resistance.[63] The huge impact on our gut microbe population[64–67] is another reason why the medical community is trying very hard to reduce antibiotic use. Our microbiome is integral to health and antibiotics have far-reaching implications that we are just beginning to realise the magnitude of. So, for now, trust your doctor's opinion and keep in mind that while you're on antibiotics it's even more important to follow my suggestions to keep your microbiome as nurtured as possible.

• Refined carbohydrates, sugars and sweeteners all have a number of links with poor health outcomes. Their effect on your microbiome is an addition to the growing list. I would exercise caution for any 'diet' versions of popular drinks and any foods with synthetic sweeteners as they can adversely affect your microbes.[68] I still use a little sugar in recipes as an ingredient to heighten flavour and taste because it's not a bad thing when used sparingly. But there are clear disadvantages to consuming it in excess, and indulgence will affect your microbiome population for the worse.[69]

• Exercise, laughter and mindfulness are not what you'd typically expect on a conventionally trained doctor's prescription pad, but it's definitely on mine! As well as the wealth of positive effects on mental health and wellbeing, daily meditation and exercise may also have a positive impact on the microbiome.[70] You don't need to wear fluorescent leggings and stare blankly into the abyss. Mindfulness is any action that quietens your inner thoughts and allows active mental rest. Try a guided meditation app, breathing exercises or simply gardening as a way of releasing inner tension and letting the mind relax.

The science examining our microbiome is accelerating at an incredible pace. I'm sure we will learn more in the coming years about how to nurture this inner population that is inseparable from our wellbeing. I truly believe that future approaches to medicine will involve a significant appreciation for 'gut health' . My recipes will show you how to keep your gut bugs happy, which will ultimately have a wealth of good effects for you.

I've written more about these lifestyle changes on my website: www.thedoctorskitchen.com

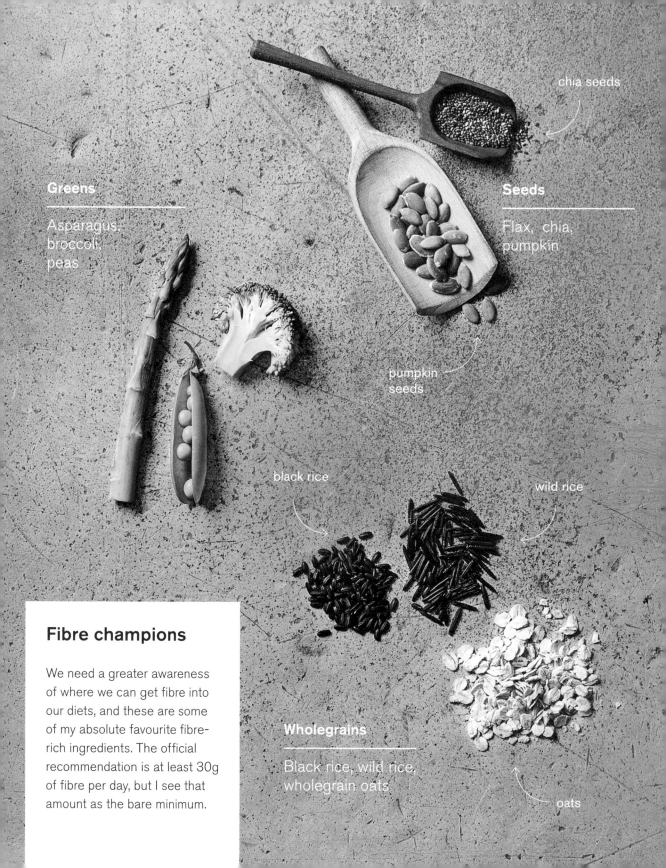

chia seeds

Greens

Asparagus,
broccoli,
peas

Seeds

Flax, chia,
pumpkin

pumpkin
seeds

black rice

wild rice

Fibre champions

We need a greater awareness
of where we can get fibre into
our diets, and these are some
of my absolute favourite fibre-
rich ingredients. The official
recommendation is at least 30g
of fibre per day, but I see that
amount as the bare minimum.

Wholegrains

Black rice, wild rice,
wholegrain oats

oats

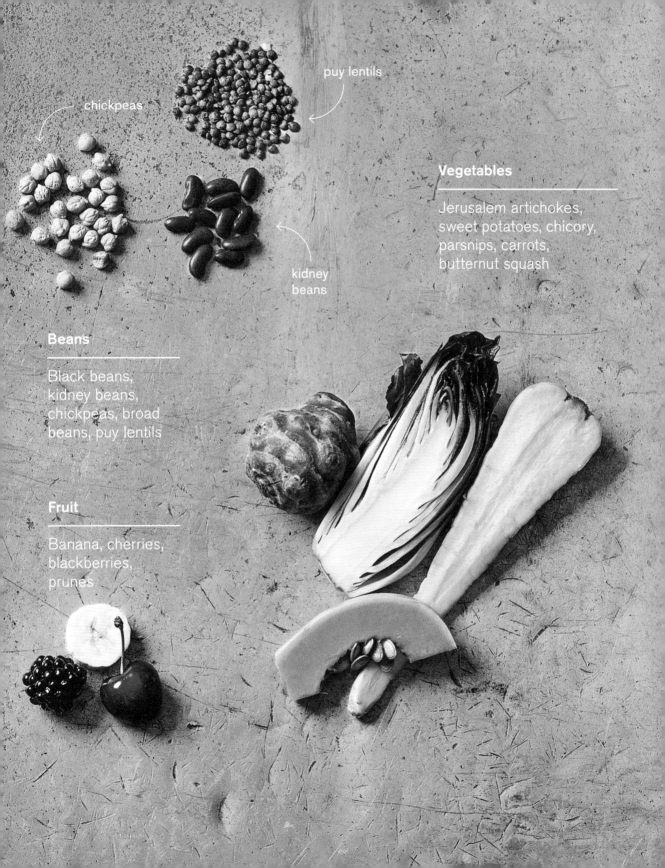

chickpeas

puy lentils

kidney beans

Vegetables

Jerusalem artichokes, sweet potatoes, chicory, parsnips, carrots, butternut squash

Beans

Black beans, kidney beans, chickpeas, broad beans, puy lentils

Fruit

Banana, cherries, blackberries, prunes

Food is information

Our culinary journey through food in medicine could not be complete without visiting the topic of how food and lifestyle affect the very foundations of our existence.

Genes, made up of DNA, are what we inherit from our parents. They are the molecular code for characteristics such as how we look, the likelihood that we will get a chronic disease and even our behavioural traits. They also regulate intricate processes in the body, such as how we deal with inflammation and remove cancer cells. Vitamins and minerals, as well as things such as sleep quality and stress, can all impact the factors that alter the expression of our genes for better, or worse, health.

What has this got to do with food? Everything.

Micronutrition and the timing of when we eat as can alter our gene expression.[71,72] Our food is constantly communicating with our DNA.

This area of research is adding yet another layer of complexity to the scientific study of why and how what we eat affects our health. There is a wealth of information available on this subject far beyond the remit of this cookbook! If you are interested, I have extra information on my website, www.thedoctorskitchen.com, including links to reading materials on subjects such as nutrigenomics, nutrigenetics and epigenetics.

Despite its complexity, I included this section because I want you to appreciate the incredible effect food has on our longevity. I want to share some insight into the fascinating studies that have framed my understanding of how food has positive effects on our bodies.[73,74] It explains why I try to weave certain ingredients into my dishes that tick the boxes for both flavour and function.

By including these delicious ingredients in our diet we can potentially affect our genetic functioning for the better.[75] Today, we can start this colourful and enjoyable journey toward good health.

I hope this motivates and inspires you to look at adapting your diet as a powerful, positive intervention. On a personal note, learning more about this field of study encouraged me to increase my intake of certain foods and explore lifestyle practices that may improve the functioning of my body. I believe that if we focus on wellness and introducing health-promoting foods and activities, the body has incredible potential to look after itself, as has been my personal experience. It's so empowering to know that despite our genes, we have the ability to steer the direction of our destiny using lifestyle.[71,76] Food is integral to this process. It is the cornerstone of healthcare and one of the biggest joys in life.

So, what do we need to eat to improve our gene functioning? In a very general sense, ensuring we have a variety of micronutrients (vitamins and minerals) is the best way to ensure proper functioning of our cells and expression of our genes. Our understanding is still basic and there's a long road ahead, but there are some key diet and lifestyle measures that we can all incorporate to ensure the correct functioning of our bodies. The good news is, these micronutrient-dense foods are tasty, cheap and easy to

Already, there are tools you can buy that can read your genetic profile and claim to give you tailored nutrition advice online, but I suggest treating these with caution. Simply looking at genetic profiling in isolation is a narrow perspective to take and it's not as simple as 'eating to beat your genes'. Health outcomes are the result of a complex interplay of food, gut health, environmental stressors and many other variables. The future of medicine is definitely personal[77] and I'm certain it will soon become the norm to have these tests, but they have to be taken in the context of the individual's circumstances. We are sophisticated machines with multiple pathways beyond our genes that we need to consider, but it doesn't stop me from getting excited about the future application of these tools for practitioners.

cook with. Here are some examples of foods I encourage my patients to eat regularly, and a snapshot of the science that explains why.

Greens for your genes

Romanesco cauliflower, cabbages of all kinds, pak choy, rocket leaves, broccoli, broccoli sprouts, Brussels sprouts, cavolo nero, kale, chard…

Everyone knows that these greens are 'good for us'. It has been drilled into our heads since childhood. But, apart from fibre and vitamins, greens have a wealth of other properties. Cruciferous vegetables (also known as brassicas), in particular, are known for their sulforaphane content. Sulforaphane is a plant chemical currently being researched for its ability to stabilise cells and protect against cancer. It also appears to impact a master regulator of genes involved in reducing cancer activity.[78]

But this is merely one of the hundreds of compounds involved in the mechanism of why

greens are 'good for us'. Cauliflower, broccoli, broccoli sprouts and rocket leaves all contain sulforaphane, plus a whole lot more that hasn't yet been fully investigated. And these vegetables don't just contain novel chemicals; they are also full of micronutrients like magnesium and folate which are vital for repairing and producing DNA.[79,80]

One of the key features of the influential Dean Ornish study[73] that showed lifestyle changes could promote genes that fight cancer, was a plant-focused diet high in cruciferous vegetables. Best of all, these ingredients can taste wonderful with the right spices, herbs and cooking techniques to moderate their naturally bitter taste. You'll want to have these affordable foods every day.

Spice your DNA

Herbs and spices are what make cooking and eating so pleasurable. In Middle Eastern cuisines, they often serve fresh herbs alongside tagines and stews to complement the rich, earthy flavours.

Vietnamese food is commonly presented with a side plate brimming with mint leaves and whole coriander stems. Our Indian version of a salad (see page 156) includes sliced red onion, fresh lemons and, of course, raw chilli. As a child, I would watch in awe as my father ate small bites of whole green chilli with his meals. I still haven't quite acquired the taste for this level of heat!

Fresh leaves are more than just sharp flavour notes to accompany a meal. Simple herbs like parsley, for example, contain plant chemicals called flavones.[81] These are known to promote the activity of genes that are responsible for suppressing inflammation,[82,83] a key feature in conditions like cancer and diabetes.

And it's not just parsley … rosemary, turmeric, ginger, oregano, onion and garlic are also abundant with health-promoting chemicals including epigalletins, quercetin, luteolin and others with equally long and confusing names.[84] To cover just our limited knowledge of all these compounds and their potential uses would fill volumes of books.

I don't want to steer you in the direction of only eating particular foods to alter your gene activity – I simply want you to appreciate the immense power of everyday ingredients. Herbs and spices are very much part of that line-up. So, when you look at my recipes, notice how highly flavoured and spiced they are. There is a method behind these flavour-packed dishes.

Colour your plate

I'm passionate about colours. They truly represent the complexity and beauty of food. Beyond their spectacular visual display and abundance of antioxidants, colourful foods are exceptionally important for us for their effects on our genes.[75] Plant chemicals (also called phytochemicals and phytonutrients) are responsible for these beautiful pigments and are usually found concentrated in the skins of fruits and vegetables.

We know that reducing inflammation is hugely important when it comes to longevity and reducing the risk of diseases ranging from dementia to depression.[85] An example of a plant chemical that gives food a vibrant, red colour is anthocyanin.[86] You'll find this in everything from beetroot and wild berries to red onion (not just pomegranate juice and acai powder!). Anthocyanins are known to activate the gene responsible for heightening antioxidant activity which can prevent against cancer.[87] It is an incredible ingredient, but one of literally thousands that could be just as impressive.

Rather than using a reductionist approach to the science that concentrates on the benefits of singular compounds, I implore you to remember that all foods have a number of chemicals in varying amounts that are wonderful.[88] Variety and nutrient density is the goal here. Don't focus too much on exact lists of ingredients and their chemical attributes. Choose vibrant colours and foods that you and your family will enjoy to reap the benefits of nature's gifts. And remember … don't throw away the skins!

The power of your microbiome

The microbiome is a feature of our health that we've already visited (see page 24). It is the name we give to the trillions of microbes (mostly bacteria) that reside all over our body but mainly in the gut. Because of the sheer number of microbes in this population, your microbiome consists of over 100 times more genetic material than your own.[89] This population has immense impact on the health of your body and mind because the microbiome genetic code is quite literally communicating and interacting with your own.[90,91] The scientific community has only started appreciating this information over the last 20 years. The most exciting feature is that although we cannot change our own genetic information, the genes and health of our microbial population can be altered by environment and that affects the expression of our DNA.[92]

This may all sound quite fantastical – the fact that our destiny is in our hands. We are quite far away from precision treatments that alter the microbiome for specific health outcomes, but science tells us that if we eat and live according to principles that help our microbiome population thrive, we live healthier lives and are less likely to suffer disease. One of the probable reasons for this is because the microbiome has an ability to positively affect the expression of our DNA.

Nurturing your gut health (see page 24) could prove vital in disease prevention and treatment.

Lifestyle for genes

• Sleep is integral to health. It's also very impactful on our microbiome and our circadian rhythms that affect our biology and gene expression.[93] Melatonin is a hormone (produced during adequate sleep) which activates and regulates hundreds of genes involved in repair, antioxidant function and, you guessed it, inflammation.[94,95] Sleep does far more than just let your muscles repair and brain recuperate; it's essential for protecting you against disease. So, practise good sleep hygiene: try not to eat or use electronic stimuli two hours before bed, and sleep your way to health.

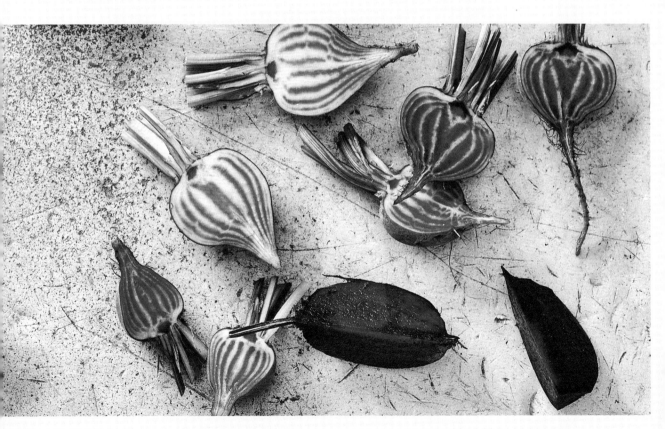

• Fasting is a practice made popular by diets like 5:2 and proponents of 'ancestral eating' that aim to mimic the lifestyles of former hunter-gatherer populations. While I take issue with blindly following a standard diet, fasting is a component of these regimes that may have some legs. Incorporating a fasting practice into your eating habits has been shown to improve the expression of genes that are responsible for removing oxidants that cause inflammation and turning on genes that fight cancer cells.[96,97] But fasting doesn't need to be a tedious feat where you remove all sources of energy for a 24-hour period. I'm a fan of defining your eating period to 10–11 hours per day. For example, if you were to eat breakfast at 8am, try not to eat dinner later than 7pm. Getting into a routine where you have the same 'defined eating period' on a daily basis may have benefits by heightening the expression of genes that control sugar and lead to greater longevity.[98,99,97] Most of the studies also found that participants lost weight and this has obviously generated a lot of attention, but in my opinion losing weight isn't necessarily always the goal. If we focus on introducing health-promoting habits and wonderful nutrition I am certain you will lose weight, but more importantly it will be enjoyable, safer and much better for your overall health. Wellness is the goal rather than a desired number on a set of scales.

• Mindfulness doesn't have to be cliché. My father grew up on a farm. He would wake up before dawn every single day and in his sleepy state make the short walk to the farm where he would duly milk the cows for the family's breakfast and butter-churning routine. This could be considered an example of mindfulness. An activity which removes thought and reason, and incorporates routine. Where the mind is quiet, restful and unstimulated.

Buddhists sweep. Beach bums surf. Commuters listen to smartphone apps. However you decide to practise it, mindfulness has never been so important as it is in now, in today's world of excessive electronic use and hyperactivity.

We live in a perpetual state of anxiety, provoked by constant stimuli, and I believe meditation is key. One of the most impressive research studies I have come across was a small experiment looking at a group of people taught to meditate over a three-week period. Using a specific gene marker to measure the inevitable ageing process, they discovered that the meditation had *improved* the marker that was expected to naturally worsen.[100,101] Meditation has been hypothesised to have a literal anti-ageing effect.[102] If an intervention can alter gene activity to that extent, it has a place as a 'medicine' in my opinion. So, decide on your meditative strategy and practise it for at least 10–20 minutes each day. You should find it has a calming effect on your mood, even if we can't conclusively prove its effect on wrinkles.

We live in a perpetual state of anxiety, provoked by constant stimuli, and I believe meditation is key.

Diet choice fatigue

I'll let you into a secret you probably already know by now: there is no such thing as a 'perfect diet'.

We are all unique as a result of our cultural backgrounds, genetic variations and even gut microbe populations. Our physical attributes are the sum of so many variables, it is unfathomable to think that any one regimen would be suitable for an entire population.

Our diets are fluid, ever-changing interactions that involve the environment and even our life cycle. The food we eat is dictated by geography, convenience and personal choices. Our nutritional needs are determined by age, hormone profile and emotional state, and that's before we even start considering medical conditions. We are complicated beings. Forcing ourselves to rigidly stick to a list of foods that are labelled 'good' or 'bad' will never reflect the intricacies of our requirements.

My goal is for you to enjoy food and appreciate the phenomenal effects it can have on your body, your mental outlook and overall health. I'm not here to scaremonger you or belittle any successes you may have had with previous experiences of diets; if you have used one of these in the past and felt better, that's fantastic! As long as you feel healthy, it fits into your lifestyle, and it doesn't lead to a nutritional deficiency or personal risk of disease, you're doing a great job. I'm not here to warn you off a way of eating that works for you and I'm very open-minded to the success of certain diets for different people. As a doctor, I just want to make sure you're safe and healthy.

If you're new to this world, I want you to understand the importance of individuality. I would rather empower you to create a unique way of eating that caters for your requirements, than suggest you follow a 'one-size-fits-all' approach.

Eating is a lifestyle, not an uncompromising 'diet'. It's a personal and experimental process that needs adapting as you and your environment change. This book, or any other book for that matter, will not contain the answer to everyone's dietary requirements. But don't despair! I've included principles of eating on page 62 that I think are applicable to most people, then the tweaking of elements really depends on you. Seek appropriate advice and get a second opinion if you have concerns about a specific medical condition.

Most diets out there promote a way of eating that is generally better than the typical Western diet of refined carbohydrates and a lack of fibre and micronutrients. So, no wonder there are so many success stories with a lot of them! This doesn't necessarily validate these diets as a way of eating for all of us. But, it's likely that you'll incorporate elements and principles from a variety of diets to create the perfect way of eating for you. Because I get asked about these in clinic all the time, I've decided to give you my opinion on the most popular diets around: the good, the bad and the science that doesn't always stack up.

Just cut the carbs!

+ Paleo, Low-carb high-fat, Atkins, South Beach, Ketogenic I know proponents of each of these diets will argue that these shouldn't be grouped together because there are slight variations between each, but for simplicity's sake, I have. Patients don't appear to differentiate between them and lately I've been hearing the same line in my surgery: 'So, Doctor, I've decided to cut out carbs. That's good, isn't it?' Well, not necessarily.

The principles of Paleo, South Beach and Atkins are quite similar. They revolve around reducing your intake of carbohydrate and replacing it with varying proportions of protein and fats, with 'low-carb high-fat' (aka LCHF) and Ketogenic diets being the most excessive in terms of fat consumption. They've been reported in clinical studies to improve markers of diabetes[103,104] and famously autoimmune disease[105] in a number of protocols. The most exciting promise for Ketogenic diets is in treating childhood epilepsy and chronic pain.[106,107]

I think these types of diets do have a place for certain people looking to re-sensitise themselves to insulin after a longstanding over-indulgence in refined carbohydrates and sugar. There is small-scale evidence to show its potential in improving diabetes, insulin sensitivity[108] and symptoms of PCOS.[109,110]

However, there is some evidence pointing toward high protein intake being similarly harmful as high carbohydrate intake, which is the trap a lot of people fall into when following these diets.[111]

And let's not forget the side effects that include: constipation, halitosis, nausea, renal stones, osteoporosis and a potentially increased risk of bowel cancer (among many others).

A lot of people can't maintain the diet for these reasons, and when they return to eating carbohydrate there appears to be a trend toward regaining all the weight they had lost with potentially worse outcomes and health risks than before they began.

On balance, long-term evidence to advocate these diets is lacking. Essentially, it's a temporary fix. I appreciate the potential therapeutic value of these diets as a short-term strategy, but personally, I think a diet concentrated on plant nutrition far outweighs one focused on meat. More research is needed to validate the claims of these diets that drastically remove beneficial carbohydrate sources, and the lack of fruit, vegetables and fibre is something that would concern me. We know fibre is essential for proper functioning of our digestive system: our microbes feed off these materials and lack of fibre puts us at risk of bowel cancer.[112] For those reasons, I can't condone low-carb lifestyles long-term, but I don't doubt that some people have found them beneficial and they may have a role in clinical care.

SIRT diet

While I welcome excitement about foods that have the potential to impact our genetic make-up, the SIRT diet's focus on a small list of foods impacting some genetic pathways detracts from how multifaceted and complicated human nutrition is. 'SIRT' genes are what this diet is named after and increasing the activity of these genes (and the proteins they code for) is thought to reduce inflammation, control blood sugar and has been linked to reducing cancer risk.[113]

Yes, parsley, dark chocolate and green tea all increase SIRT gene expression but they also contain catechins, luteolin and a host of micronutrients that are essential for processes in our body's cells. As do lupini beans, cavolo nero, broccoli, coriander, chilli and a whole bunch of foods that don't fit a particular list. I think it completely misses the point to focus on an exclusive group of ingredients, and it doesn't encourage a healthy relationship with food. Every ingredient deserves a platform.

Our grocery aisles are lined with unbelievable health-promoting foods, our seasons provide constant variety and our multicultural society introduces spices and herbs from across the planet. As I alluded to in the previous section, we are merely scratching the surface when it comes to the importance of different interactions between ingredients and our genes. I could have quite easily picked out a few fruits, vegetables and spices affecting one of many inflammatory pathways and called it the 'NRF2 diet', or how about the 'TNF diet'? The Telomere diet? Do these sound scientifically valid enough?

The interaction between food and our genetics is a fascinating field.[114] But it is one layer of a multi-faceted process that I haven't made the cavalier attempt of trying to explain in its entirety. It certainly cannot be explained with one set of genes. Don't let yourselves be patronised. Our understanding of these pathways is minuscule at best[115] … and don't get me started on 'juice cleanses'!

The interaction between food and our genetics is a fascinating field.

5:2 diet

The science used to formulate intermittent fasting diets like the 5:2 diet is impressive.[116] There appear to be benefits of cyclical fasting,[117,118] but our way of eating needs to be sustainable[119] and more importantly, enjoyable. Who wants to endure restricting themselves on a weekly basis … for life? I am convinced that some people have found benefits from this practice,[120] but if I were to tell the majority of patients I see in clinic to reduce their calories to 500 for two whole days, I know exactly where they'd be telling me to go!

And this brings me nicely to another topic. I don't count calories. For the majority of people it's a complete waste of time because it shifts the focus toward indiscriminate numbers on packets of food and away from what is actually important: the quality of food we introduce into our body. Clearly, a bag of sugar compared to an equal calorie content of spinach is going to have drastically different effects on our body. Calorie counting does not account for this difference. It focuses unnecessarily on a logic that was once thought to be scientifically accurate but is now shown to be flawed in many ways.

+ A NOTE ON CALORIES

The long-held idea that excessive calorie consumption leads to weight gain and reducing calories leads to weight loss is simply not accurate. Also, the metabolism of food is likely to differ from person to person depending on a host of factors such as their microbiome population, their genes, activity level, timing of meals and many other variables. A 200-calorie lunch isn't necessarily 'healthier' than the 500-calorie one, and two identical calorie meals can have entirely different metabolic effects. The majority of people I see in clinic do not need to diligently measure and obsess about these numbers.

When we encourage concentrating on calories, or even the Glycaemic Index (GI) of foods, we lose sight of the bigger picture. People find themselves picking up ready-made desserts and putting down bananas. This is madness. There is a huge difference between the metabolic effect of packaged meals and a whole food. Diets that promote this are not educative and they serve to confuse rather than inspire, with dire consequences. Relax, cook as often as possible at home using whole ingredients, and put the calorie counters away.

Fasting, and the variations of fasting practices[120], is an interesting area and warrants further research. But, what I think is potentially as effective and easier to incorporate into daily working life is the concept of defined eating periods.[121] A time period during the day when you eat versus a period when you do not eat. Research also shows that the simple effort of ensuring you eat at regular times and within a 10–11-hour window can reduce your risk of diabetes and cardiovascular disease.[122] It stabilises insulin release and leads to less fat around the organs (which is dangerous). It makes logical sense to me and a lot of my patients are easily able to slot this convenient 'fasting' practice into their eating habits that doesn't require obsessive calorie counting or restriction.

Alkaline diet

I'm going to give you some insight as to why there is such a divide between physicians and the wellness industry. When non-medically trained, self-styled, health 'gurus' are given a platform to influence people into believing they can change their blood pH with a diet high in alkaline foods, it is incredibly frustrating. You can change the pH of your urine using food, but the suggestion that this diet has a miraculous, transformational total-body effect is a huge oversimplification of the science.[123]

Fundamentally, this diet encourages us to eat more dark green leafy vegetables and generally healthier foods, which isn't a bad thing.[124,125] However, people deserve to be educated and told the truth about how food interacts with our biochemistry, instead of being duped into thinking this is how our bodies work. When you've spent time in intensive care, learnt about the complexities of acid-base balance in

ill patients and tried to get your head around how complicated pH control is,[126,127] you can understand why the use of alkaline theories to promote products annoy doctors all round. We have intelligently evolved organs that precisely control our blood pH using mechanisms that still continue to amaze me.

Introducing 'alkaline' foods such as brassica vegetables and colourful fruits is fantastic, but rather than just focusing on 'alkalinity', we should appreciate the phytochemical content, the fibre and micronutrients like folate and magnesium. We also need to consider the relatively low sugar content and the endless chemicals that we haven't yet fully investigated. Focusing on 'alkalinity' confuses the matter and I fear it will create an obsession among patients akin to calorie counting. I am an open-minded doctor, so perhaps one day we will learn more about 'alkalinity', but for now the science just does not support these claims.[128,123,129] I would have great reservations for the liberal use of these ideas, especially by those who cannot appreciate the scientific controversy.

Low Fat/Slimming World/ NHS Choices

The medical profession's obsession with reducing the fat content of our food and encouraging processed, low-fat options over the past few decades has probably been the most effective, yet destructive, health campaign of all time. It's a message I myself have been guilty of promoting. An over-indulgence in calories, particularly from fat, combined with apathy toward exercise was the generally accepted explanation for why patients were overweight and sick. It was arrogant and naïve to accept this assumption that gluttony was the underlying cause of patients' illnesses and not question its legitimacy. It's obvious, now, that this was not correct.[130,131]

Hydrogenated fats, 'cholesterol-lowering' products and sugar-laden alternatives that we promoted are terrible options for the vulnerable cohort of patients we were trying to help.[132–135] The recommendations for extreme restriction of saturated fat, cholesterol and total fat are now becoming obsolete and further analysis is proving fat not to be as detrimental to health as we once thought.[136,137] The morbid result of our fixation with replacing fats with refined carbohydrates and sugar is exemplified by our current lifestyle-related disease epidemic.[138]

However, the restricted fat message still exists, particularly among supporters of plant-based lifestyles. To their credit, some small studies demonstrate remarkable cardiovascular disease reversal and cancer improvement using fat restriction and lifestyle change.[139,73] On the other hand, the Mediterranean diet, one of the largest and longest studied of eating habits, comprises three times more fat than 'fat-restricted' diets with – again – impressive cardiovascular, cancer and diabetes protective effects.[50,48]

My honest opinion is that we shouldn't fear fat. We don't exactly know why some people thrive on low fat intake while others suffer, but I'm certain it comes down to the individual.[140] Your environment, gut microbes and ancestry play a major role in predicting the success of any given diet and lowering your risk of disease, but I believe a good proportion of good-quality fats are essential to health.

+ RETHINKING FATS

Fats, including cholesterol, are vital to the functioning of our brains, the composition of cell structures and essential for hormone synthesis. Reducing them to 'good' and 'bad' fats completely negates the science and lacks an appreciation for how complicated our bodies are. My belief is that a high-sugar, refined-carbohydrate diet in combination with poor-quality fats is the cause of ill health.[141] This toxic blend causes inflammation and a cascade of medical problems thereafter, but like a lot of topics in nutrition, the explanation is fraught with complexity. Our thinking about how dietary cholesterol affects heart disease is also changing.[142,143,144] Consuming cholesterol, which is only found in animal products, does not necessarily increase the level of cholesterol found in your blood nor increase your risk of heart disease. I know this is quite hard for a lot of people to accept, given the dietary dogma most of us have been subjected to over the last 40 years, but it is based on evidence. Equally, I don't recommend people actively try to consume more cholesterol. We need to learn from our past mistakes of damning an entire macronutrient to the extent that people are scared into radically removing it, but what I am witnessing now is a swing of the metaphorical pendulum in the opposite direction! Even though butter has been exonerated to some degree, you won't find me spooning it into my coffee – I like my Americano freshly brewed without lipid-rich particles floating in it, thank you very much.

For simplicity's sake, I stick to the types of fats found in the Mediterranean diet which is packed with nuts, seeds and, of course, extra-virgin olive oil. My simple mantra to patients is: eat whole food and stay away from anything that's marketed as 'low fat' or 'a healthier alternative to …' Your body is worth more than those cheap, tasteless alternatives. Some quality fats to enjoy in the context of a whole-foods diet include those found in flaxseeds, nuts, seeds, avocado, extra-virgin olive oil, butter from grass-fed cows, full-fat yoghurt and delicious dark chocolate.

Veganism

In recent times plant-based eating has become exceptionally popular. A number of documentaries have convinced many people of the supposed health benefits of veganism and the health risks of red meat. They do have a lot of successes to feel smug about, that are well documented in the literature. Lower rates of cancer,[145] diabetes,[146] cardiovascular disease[147]… the list goes on. It's compelling stuff and, obviously, I'm a huge supporter of a diet largely made up of fruits and vegetables, but pure veganism doesn't come without its caveats. B vitamins are noticeably lacking in vegans, as well as zinc, essential fatty acids and vitamin D.[148] Careful supplementation with extra nutrients is something I would advise all 100-per-cent plant-based eaters to discuss with their health practitioner.

Also, it's important to remember that just because you go vegan doesn't automatically turn you into a dementia-proof, cancer-kicking superhuman with spotless arteries. If I lived on chips and pasta with tomato sauce I could feel pretty ethically minded about not having killed an animal for my dinner, but I probably wouldn't live for very long to tell people about it.

Ultimately, I have a deep respect for those who choose to live a life on plants alone, whatever their reasons, but my priority would be to make sure everyone is doing it safely.

Wrapping up

What a lot of these diets have in common is a focus on weight loss as a positive outcome, but is this what we should be striving for? Is weight management a reliable biomarker of general health and should this be the common denominator against which we judge the success of a diet? BMI is such a poor predictor of outcomes yet many studies continue to use this as a standard.[149]

Everyone has the ability to lose weight, tone up and feel lighter, but sometimes it's at the expense of health rather than in pursuit of it. I want you to feel 'well'. I'm convinced that good health, contrary to popular belief, is independent of size and especially weight.[150] I think we could all do with a little less emphasis on weight as an outcome and more of a focus on wellbeing. Health and wellness conjure images of slim, vivacious, young 20-somethings, but a focus on this as the ultimate goal detracts from why we are trying to achieve a healthier life. I believe it is for the sum of our daily interactions to be positive in mind and physicality. It is to live a fulfilling and happy life. This doesn't necessarily correspond to a certain

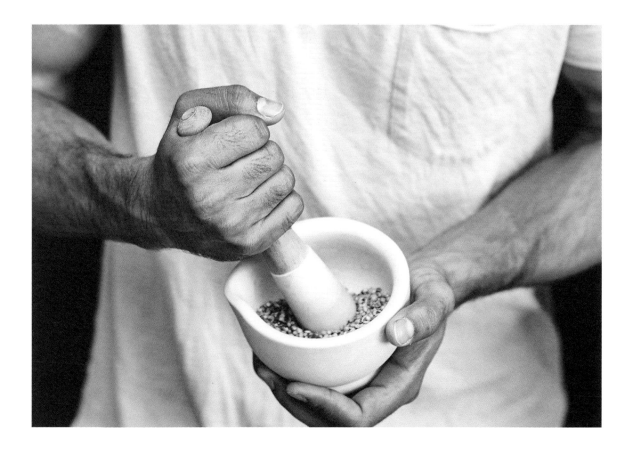

number on a machine, even though an industry, and perhaps even your doctor, is trying to convince you it does. Your focus should be on health goals and habits rather than a physical endpoint.

There are endless ways in which you can add nutrient-dense foods to your diet on a daily basis and I want to encourage people to think along these lines. We have an opportunity to be truly nourished, rather than skip from diet to diet in the hope that we hit the 'carb-protein-fat ratio jackpot' and achieve that dazzling 'perfect weight'.

I'm convinced that good health, contrary to popular belief, is independent of size and especially weight.

Growing up in an Indian household, I was constantly surrounded by spices, herbs and folk medicines. Everything from sore throats to constipation seemed treatable with the contents of our kitchen cupboards!

Most second-generation kids will concur: Indian families seem to have an encyclopaedic knowledge for complementary health cures. I have vivid memories of being fed a spoonful of toasted spices and salt whenever I had tummy ache. My father would always make a mixture of almonds, clarified butter and sugar during my exams, claiming it was 'brain food'. And, of course, my mother was years ahead of the 'Spiced Turmeric Latte' trend.

You can imagine the number of 'I told you so's' I got when I started researching the clinical validity of traditional treatments. My Indian heritage is steeped in Ayurvedic tradition and what fascinates me is the premise of 'alternative therapies' having the potential to become recognised treatment in the battle against chronic disease. Learning about the marriage of flavour and medicinal property was revolutionary for me.

The positive clinical effects of food are unlikely to be caused by a single ingredient, like a spice or herb, so it's important to maintain a holistic perspective. Remember that any benefit from the inclusion of an ingredient has to be taken in the context of a 'good diet'. Reiterating what I stated at the start of this book: **do not treat food like a pill.** Concoctions from herbalists or 'natural' food supplements are not panaceas or cure-alls, in exactly the same way that anti-diabetic

medications will not manage a patient's condition if they don't make changes in their lifestyle to complement treatment. Nonetheless, this does not stop me getting excited about the incredible effects of spices.

Spices make food visibly enticing by adding colour and enhancing the flavour and aroma of the most uninspiring ingredients. Using precise techniques, we can quantify their high antioxidant capacity and activity, which explains why we've used spice as a preservative for centuries. There is enough evidence to support the daily inclusion of nature's wonderful spices and here are some staples I believe everyone should have in the store cupboard and the clinical evidence as to why.

Turmeric

Turmeric is probably one of the most extensively researched spices we have in nutritional science and it's now commonly accepted that daily dietary inclusion can prevent bowel cancer. There's also evidence that it could be beneficial for helping dementia, chronic pain syndromes and inflammatory conditions.[151] It's astonishing what effects a single ingredient can potentially have on the body.

As is usually the case in nutritional therapy, supplementation using high doses of one of

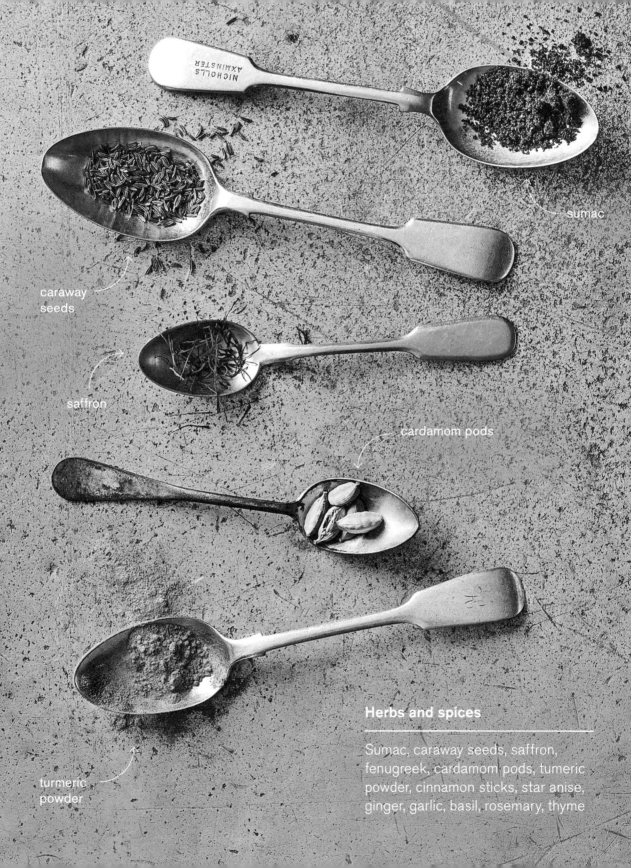

sumac

caraway
seeds

saffron

cardamom pods

turmeric
powder

Herbs and spices

Sumac, caraway seeds, saffron,
fenugreek, cardamom pods, tumeric
powder, cinnamon sticks, star anise,
ginger, garlic, basil, rosemary, thyme

NICHOLLS AXMINSTER

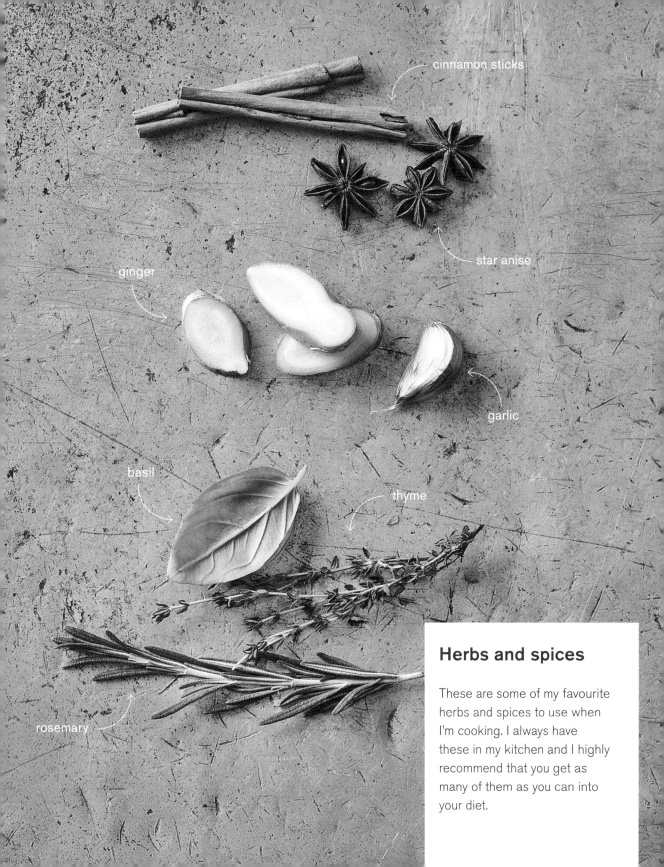

cinnamon sticks

star anise

ginger

garlic

basil

thyme

rosemary

Herbs and spices

These are some of my favourite herbs and spices to use when I'm cooking. I always have these in my kitchen and I highly recommend that you get as many of them as you can into your diet.

turmeric's active compounds, 'curcumin', has had mixed results.[152,153] Turmeric is not just curcumin. The spice is made up of hundreds of different plant chemicals of which curcumin is just one. These studies teach us a lesson: use *whole* plants as much as possible rather than isolated chemicals. A single component is not likely to be responsible for their health benefits; it's the complex arrangement of molecules in whole ingredients that we find in nature.

I use ground turmeric in everything from Malaysian curry pastes to soups and stews; and if you can get hold of the fresh stuff that looks like ginger with bright orange flesh, even better. Using fresh turmeric in cooking with other ingredients like chilli and black pepper (that contain capsaicin and piperine) heightens its effect and availability in the body.[154] If nothing else gets you interested in 'food as medicine', this herbaceous plant from the ginger family should.

Garlic

I've been raised to expect garlic to be used in most dishes cooked at home. But even now, whether I'm cooking Italian, Chinese or Moroccan food, garlic forms the flavour base for most of my meals. Enough research has been published for me to believe that it can lower your risk of cancer, and laboratory studies demonstrate its anti-bacterial and anti-viral properties.[155–158] It may have a positive impact on human gut microbe populations[159,160] too, and it's so easy to incorporate into meals. It's definitely an ingredient I get into my food on a daily basis (you'll notice how often it's used in my recipes).

Garlic is also so versatile. You can simply cut the top off a whole bulb, drizzle it with olive oil and roast it for 20 minutes, squeezing the cooked pulp out of its papery skins and storing it in the fridge. I use it as a spread or flavour enhancer when making quick meals. Look out for fresh, smoked garlic and my current favourite, black garlic: it has a sweet balsamic vinegary taste and is a wonder ingredient in pesto and sauces.

Ginger

Here's another spice often used in Indian cooking, with a host of studies examining its effect on everything from cancer prevention to nausea.[161,162] Gingerols, shagoals and zingerones are all antioxidants thought to be responsible for its health effects.[163] I use fresh ginger as much as possible for its pungent taste and powerful volatile compounds. It's a staple base for lots of my recipes and sometimes I'll boil some up with honey to treat a sore throat. There are many innovative ways to use ginger in drinks, tonics, sauces and curries. My recipes will show you how easy it is to get this marvellous spice into your system.

There are well recognised polyphenol compounds in ginger and it's been suggested in the research that we class it as a functional food because of its effects on the body. I use it in my Medicinal Broth (see page 152), I pop ginger skin into tea, I grate it into Asian-style dressings (see page 252) and it's cheap and available to everyone. Get it into your kitchen.

Sumac

This vibrant burgundy-coloured spice has the most wonderful, warm citrus flavour. It's used in Iranian and Turkish cuisines in tagines and stews or simply to garnish plates with a sour note. It also happens to be one of the most antioxidant-rich ingredients on the planet.[164,165] It's been used in traditional medicine to treat everything from diabetes[166] to cardiac disease, but unfortunately the extent of research we currently have to support these claims is mainly performed in a petri dish or on animals.[167] The research is one to watch.[168]

Made from drying a species of the plant genus Rhus, sumac is generally underutilised in cooking, but I use it all the time for its incredible flavour profile and vibrancy. A sprinkle will transform everything from poached eggs to natural yoghurt. Try it out in some of my Middle Eastern-inspired dishes (see Persian Chicken Thighs on page 178, and Spicy Baked Eggs on page 77).

Cumin

Cumin is a functional spice that contains myriad compounds thought to be anti-bacterial and blood-sugar regulating (among many other claims of traditional medicine).[169] Unfortunately, again, there are not many human clinical trials examining the exact effect of this spice and when there are, they're not conducted well.[170] What we do know is that it contains a really high antioxidant capacity as well as particular compounds that have been implicated in reducing inflammation and fighting cancer.[169,171,172]

I couldn't cook without cumin (or 'jeera', as it's known in my kitchen). Used as ground seeds or whole seeds, it has an assertive taste that is distinctly Indian in my mind, but is very easily incorporated into a variety of dishes. Use it to transform your roast dinners, spice up your omelette or add an exotic hint to any meal. And, if you use it frequently, buy a bag of it from your local Indian store, not a thimble-sized jar!

Cinnamon

Another aromatic, antioxidant-packed, flavour bomb. The compounds in cinnamon have been investigated in order to explain why this spice has anti-inflammatory effects and improves metabolic syndrome.[173] Study after study reports potential mechanisms of action, and the biology, for someone interested in why spices have medicinal benefits, is groundbreaking. Reading some of the texts is like going back into pharmacology lectures at medical school. It's a fascinating field of research that I hope will unravel more information, but for now, experiment with cinnamon in my spices, dressings and pastes (see pages 240–9) to elevate simple dishes.

Its versatility permeates through savoury and sweet dishes, drinks and dressings, modern European cuisine to rural Indian meals. It's no wonder cinnamon used to be more valuable than gold in Egyptian times. Invest in a large, high-quality tub of it – you cannot have a kitchen without this spice.

Basil, rosemary, thyme

The incredible health properties of herbs and spices are not exclusive to those shipped in from the Far East or Africa. We have some amazing flavour enhancers that are easy to grow here in the UK in a pot in the kitchen, and that have as much functional benefit as the most expensive and beautiful saffron from Iran.

Basil, rosemary and thyme may seem unassuming, but the library of chemicals held within their leaves is inspiring. At the average 'doses' that we tend to use in cooking, they contain exceptionally important dietary sources of chemicals that reduce oxidative stress and attenuate inflammation.[174] The theories of heightened inflammation and its role in lifestyle-related disease, such as blood pressure, stroke and diabetes, is very fashionable in medical conferences these days.[175] Any inclusion of foods that can reduce our inflammatory burden is welcome, and these delicious, cheap, widely available herbs are worth every stalk.[176]

Adding roughly chopped basil to Italian recipes adds an extra depth of flavour. Thyme,

Any inclusion of foods that can reduce our inflammatory burden are welcome, and these delicious, cheap, widely available herbs are worth every stalk.

perhaps one of the first herbs to be recognised for its medicinal qualities, is in everything, from my fresh barbecue rubs (see page 243) to my twist on shakshuka (see page 77). Pestos, marinades, green curry pastes, aioli … the options are limitless and, as a doctor, I cannot recommend highly enough that you include these herbs in your daily diet.

Seeing past the herb garden

We really need to start investigating spice compounds further. We know that they are safe for consumption because we've essentially been testing them by including them in our diets for years,[177] and exciting early research suggests a potential role for their use in treating different conditions.[22] Don't get too fixated on the exact amounts of antioxidants or measurements of compounds in an individual spice. First, not all the evidence looks at specific 'dosing' of ingredients, and second, they have varying effects in our body. The best advice is to consume a complement of different herbs and spices daily. Their synergistic effects have been shown to heighten their physiological properties,[173] as well as adding a delicious complexity to food.

These are some of my favourite spices, but it's by no means an exhaustive list. I've also written a section on spice combinations in the recipes section (see pages 240–5) to help you get creative. Label your own spice blends – it'll impress your friends and help get kids into the kitchen!

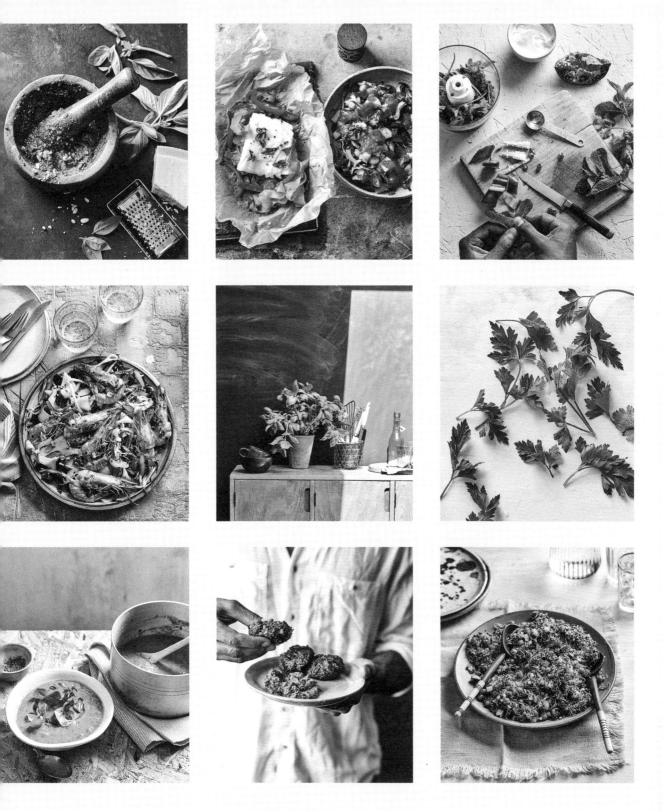

49   Introduction

Worth the extra spend?

Patients often ask me whether they should spend money on 'health foods'.

I'm encouraged by the fact that more people are interested in food, experimenting with different ingredients and at least attempting to live healthier lives, but the 'superfood' trend has its downsides. It has tainted the image of organic as something only attainable for conscientious middle classes, and perusing the aisles of 'health' sections in major supermarkets, you can forgive people for thinking eating well is costly. Some ingredients that caught media attention in recent years are incredibly expensive, and are backed by 'research' which is questionable in a lot of cases. I often get asked 'which ones are worth the money'?

As a foodie, I've probably tried most of them. But, importantly, I judge them on the evidence base of their supposed health benefits as well as their taste. If we choose to spend an exorbitant amount of money on these ingredients, they'd better be worthwhile! Bitter gourd juice has been shown to improve glucose control in diabetics, but the taste is frightful! And I can't see Western palates taking to 'Amla' powder any time soon.

However, the following 'health' ingredients, add flavour and texture and I believe are worth the extra pounds on your weekly shopping bill.

Hemp seeds

These are one of the most concentrated sources of plant-based protein available. The seeds have a whopping amount of fibre and a great fatty acid profile to make them a potentially heart-health-promoting product.[178,179] The Omega-3 fatty acids they contain are an important source of fats for largely plant-based eaters like myself.[178]

The nutty and slight oily texture of the seeds makes them a great addition to smoothies or granola, and toasted with spices they make an awesome salad topper. The seeds are easier on your digestion than most processed protein powders and far more nutritionally dense.[180] In fact, I don't use protein powders any more in my post-workout smoothies because shelled hemp seeds are brilliant and, on balance, much cheaper than those outrageously large tubs I used to buy.

Cacao powder

Raw cocoa beans are roasted and ground to create this bitter, antioxidant- and flavanol-rich product that I use in everything from Mexican Mole (see page 161) to vegan ice cream. Most people aren't aware of its incredible amino acid profile. It's a complete protein (i.e. it contains all nine essential amino acids) and its phytochemical profile is off the charts![181] It's thought to potentially reduce the risk of stroke,[182] elevate mood by preventing tryptophan destruction[183] (an amino acid used in synthesis of the neurotransmitter serotonin) and improve cardiac function by increasing nitric oxide levels in the blood.[184] It is even suggested that cacao has a positive effect in neurocognitive disorders like dementia,[185] but while I welcome this fascination surrounding polyphenol-rich foods, I wouldn't get too overexcited. Cacao may have potential applications in the future of medicine, but for now, let's focus on its culinary uses!

Once you know how to use cacao, it becomes worth the expense, and since the 'drink of gods' has become so popular, it has also become a lot cheaper! The lengthy process of making the raw powder justifies its price, and the depth of flavour it offers makes it a worthwhile purchase. Look for 100 per cent powder, not cocoa with added dried milk products and sugar. Follow some of my simple recipes (see pages 161 and 234) to discover how versatile it is in both savoury and sweet dishes and acquire the taste for this wonderful ingredient. You can get the same nutritional benefits from using high-quality dark chocolate powder, which I don't think I could live without (75 per cent cocoa solids or higher is ideal).

Quinoa

I still get some eye rolling when I mention quinoa to my colleagues! But quinoa in all its coloured varieties is a really worthwhile addition to your diet. It's good value and widely available, it's easy to cook and it has a better nutritional profile than rice, bread or pasta (higher in protein, with more vitamins and minerals[186]), plus we even produce some right here in the UK! It contains all essential amino acids and the dark varieties possess even more antioxidants than the white.

It has been labelled as a potential 'functional food', because it may help reduce the incidence of high blood pressure, metabolic syndrome and stroke.[187] This is quite a claim to make, given the lack of human studies testing these theories,[188] but is certainly an area to watch.

Note, however, that these potential benefits don't extend to every product just because it has quinoa in it. If a chocolate bar has some sprinkled puffed quinoa grains on top, this does not automatically make it a protein-rich, blood-pressure-reducing functional food! I recommend cooking with whole quinoa, and using it in both savoury and sweet dishes.

Extra-virgin olive oil

A cornerstone of the Mediterranean diet, the popularity of this polyphenol-rich fat has fluctuated in recent years, as it has found itself caught up in the battle of opinion on what constitutes a healthy plate, but I use good-quality olive oil liberally.

In the context of a low-sugar, nutrient-dense diet, olive oil has been shown to potentially be protective of heart health[189] and, importantly, makes food so much more enjoyable. 'EVOO', as it's affectionately called by health bloggers, is thought to reduce oxidative stress because of its good fatty acid content[190] and rich diversity of phenolics.[191] The role of oxidation and inflammation in heart disease has become well recognised in the medical community, so it's probably the antioxidant effect of EVOO that makes it a heart-healthy ingredient.

It's a staple in my store cupboard and fat of choice for lightly sautéing food, dressing dishes and making pestos. It remains stable (the chemical bonds do not break down) up to reasonable cooking temperatures around 170°C[192] and the difference in taste between poor- and high-quality EVOO is noticeable to even the least refined of palates. Spend a few extra pounds on organic, cold-pressed[193] olive oil – your heart will thank you for it.

Matcha

Matcha is a finely ground powder made from green tea leaves. I hesitated to include it because I appreciate it is an expensive product, but the evidence on its dual role in both cancer prevention and helping those undergoing cancer treatment is really interesting.[194] Its high consumption in Japan is thought to be one of a multitude of reasons why they have such low cancer rates.[195] Study after study also reports benefits for cardiovascular disease, diabetes and – most notably – improving cognition.[196,197] It seems like there's nothing green tea can't be good for!

Most studies have tried to isolate specific compounds like the ECGC (epigallocatechin-gallate) responsible for matcha's health effects,[198] but don't let this reductionist science confuse you. Just like in the case of curcumin found in turmeric (see page 43), the health effects of green tea are likely due to the sum of many different chemicals that it is composed of rather than an individual one. It contains one of the richest and varied sources of polyphenols of any ingredient and the beneficial effects are seen when it's consumed in its whole form. Rather than taking a supplement of one of its chemicals, enjoy a cup of green tea the traditional way.

It's incredibly versatile to use, but only buy matcha if you actually enjoy its earthy taste. You can use it in all kinds of creative ways: in sweet creams, desserts (see page 221) or as a tea simply served alongside a Japanese meal. Personally, I find the slow ceremony of making

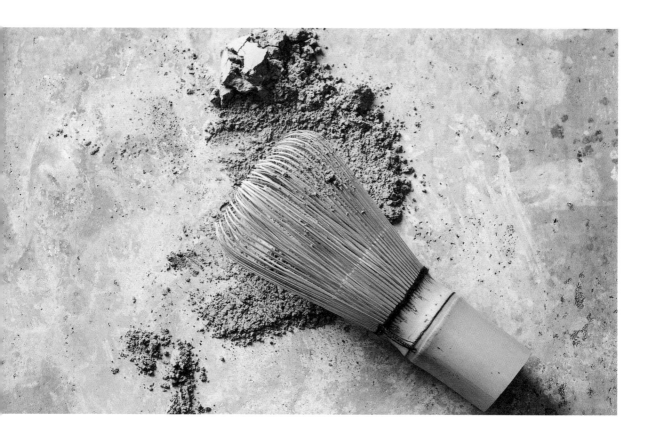

matcha tea the traditional way, using a bamboo whisk, quite calming and therapeutic. Give it a try!

Flaxseeds/Linseeds

The flax trend is definitely in full swing. You can find it packed into brownies, granolas, and many other foods to which it adds its nutty taste. I love it. Like shelled hemp seed, it's a great source of Omega-3 fats[199] and fibre, and it's full of protein.[200] There are some small studies that demonstrate its positive effect on glucose control,[201] but like most foods, more research is needed to prove any of these claims, due to a lack of human clinical trials. For now, it's an all-round nutritious ingredient that I use in everything from smoothies to my Meatless Meatballs (see page 204).

Berries

Most of us are aware of the antioxidant punch that dark berries offer. The multiple different phytochemicals, such as anthocyanins, that give rise to their beautiful pigments, have heart-protective effects,[202] may shield against dementia[203,204] and are implicated in why certain populations live longer on average.[205] Fresh berries are often the most expensive fruit on the shelves, but frozen berries are much cheaper and sufficiently hold their nutritional value. Red cabbage, purple broccoli, sweet potato, red onion and cherries are examples of different ingredients that have a similar phytochemical content to berries. Dried exotic berries such as barberries, are great, too, plus gooseberries and cranberries which can be cheap, are low in sugar and have protective properties. When berries are in season they are much cheaper, so stock up your freezer in the summer months!

Try and opt for whole berries rather than dehydrated and powdered versions. The process of heating berries, grinding them down to a powder and exposing a greater surface area of the fruit to oxygen drastically reduces their original nutrient content.[206] I throw fresh or frozen berries into smoothies and ice cream mixtures (see pages 228–30), and make them into tart sauces to pour over delicious, dark, flavanol-rich chocolate. They are perfect accompaniments and a delightful, health-promoting treat we should all indulge in.

Seaweed

Fresh samphire is actually not that pricey, but knowing where to look for it is usually the problem. You can usually find fresh varieties from your fishmonger really cheaply and slightly more expensive dried seaweed made into pastas are also available in supermarkets these days.

A staple of their cuisine, the Japanese eat seaweed by the kilo![207] Studies of the chemical properties of seaweed have found its mineral content is incredibly high.[208] No wonder the Japanese age less rapidly and have lower rates of chronic disease. I believe marine plants are something we really should start acquiring the taste for – for our health's sake – even if we just serve them as a garnish. If you're new to marine plants, start with varieties of seaweed found in the UK (your local fishmonger will be able to advise you). I add fresh or dried versions to miso broth and little amounts to classic stews to give them an umami sensation!

Along with 'health' and 'super' foods, there is currently a real trend for eating SLO: seasonal, local and organic.

Proponents of eating SLO paint this beautiful picture of how we have developed alongside our environment and that our biology is intertwined with the changing produce according to its availability throughout the year. As a nomadic race, we would move according to seasons and thrive off what the land would offer.[209] It's only very recently in our evolution that we became settlers who grew crops and made more efficient use of the earth, leading to the expansion of our population.

Seasonal eating gives us a fantastic history lesson in the way we have evolved to eat food, but as the majority of us only have access to a local supermarket, it's not realistic to suggest we should all eat this way. I would rather encourage you to select a range of different fruits and vegetables, that may have been imported and accumulated food miles, than advise eating completely SLO. I don't want any of you to shy away from buying healthy produce for fear of it not being in season.

However, I do think seasonal eating is a good reminder to introduce new foods onto our plates throughout the year and encourages variety. Changing up your ingredients, as we have discussed, is what our gut microbiome thrives on, and seasonal produce tends to be cheaper, too. There's a good reason chefs aim to cook with seasonal produce – it's more flavourful. We know phytochemicals are responsible for smell, pigment and taste, so there could be functional reasons to eating seasonally.[210] The beneficial plant chemicals may be slightly higher in fruits

and vegetables when they're in season, so I always advise patients to stock up. Not just because they could be marginally better for you, but because they taste brilliant. Local produce is also probably better because it has been harvested more recently which retains more nutrients and fewer preservatives are used.[211,212]

I am a supporter of organic growing methods, but all things considered this is more down to my personal feelings about social and environmental responsibility rather than hard evidence that organically grown produce is more nutritious. The current research is not as black and white as I would hope it to be: some studies have shown little to no difference in vitamin and mineral concentrations between organic and non-organic produce. On the flip side, the compounds that give plants their disease-fighting ability are found in higher quantities in organic produce.[213] This functional aspect is key for me.

Aside from the nutritional differences, we also need to consider the use of agricultural chemicals in conventional produce. The effects of pesticides on gut health, cancer and chronic disease are ill documented and, according to most government bodies, there are not yet enough epidemiological studies to conclusively prove their negative effects.[214] However, I'm personally risk averse when it comes to the potential harmful effects of modern-day, large-scale agricultural practices, which is why – along with my understanding of the functional aspect – I choose organic where possible. I also believe that with our significant buying power as a collective population we can shape the future of our food landscape making local, organic produce cheap and available to everyone.

Inorganic versus organic is an important discussion we need to have, but don't be overwhelmed by irrational scaremongering and mixed messages. Yes, some farming compounds have been shown to be toxic, cancer-causing and detrimental on a range of levels and we should be much more careful before exposing our population without sufficient long-term safety studies.[215–217] But, there is a bigger picture. Our bodies are incredible and resilient machines. Our organs have powerful inbuilt 'detoxing' abilities, which allow us to live in smog-filled cities and tolerate the huge amounts of pollutants we're exposed to on a daily basis. The best way to support our robust structures is to flood them with a variety of produce necessary for their function and we can do this by eating colourful plant foods.

As a working doctor, foodie and health influencer it's my responsibility to be honest and representative. I do not exclusively eat organic produce. Although I prefer organic, it does not stop me ordering food in a restaurant, eating at a friend's house or out and about. Working on late shifts I find myself navigating small supermarkets and rustling up quick dinners late at night which are definitely not SLO! Unless you live on or near a farm, you too are going to be buying and eating produce out of season, non-local and inorganic. Don't be overwhelmed by SLO – it's not a fixed rule of how we should eat.[218] A matter more pressing in our current health climate is introducing the right types of food onto our plates. Utilise the principles of healthy living I introduce later in the book (see pages 62–3) and you'll be on the right track.

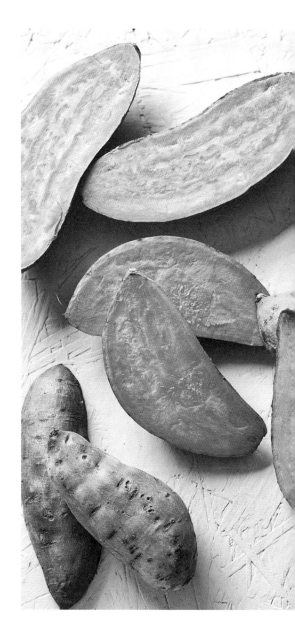

Introduction

The great gluten debate

It seems everyone is on the gluten-bashing bandwagon these days!

There are many reasons why someone would choose to go gluten free and I've realised people are in fact becoming more educated about what gluten is and why some people experience intolerance. However, there are still many misconceptions about gluten.

A quick refresher. Gluten is a mixture of two proteins (glutenin and gliadin) found in grains such as wheat and barley. It's responsible for the incredible elastic, sticky nature of bread dough that makes proper pizza crust and sourdough so delicious and chewy. Unfortunately, it's a reaction to these proteins that can cause a disease known as Coeliac Disease. This severe autoimmune disorder is characterised by damage to the lining of a patient's digestive tract causing malabsorption and pain. We diagnose Coeliac Disease using blood tests and a telescope test, known as endoscopy, to examine the intestines and take biopsies.

Traditionally, we've dismissed how gluten could possibly be related to a patient's symptoms in the absence of positive tests. If your bloods and guts look normal, it's not gluten that's causing the problem, right? However, a huge grey area dubbed 'Non Coeliac Gluten Sensitivity' is now becoming well recognised in the scientific community,[219,220] following the work of Harvard Medical School Professor Alessio Fasano.[221,222] He's responsible for discovering a particular protein within gut cells that causes microscopic damage and intestinal permeability (also called 'leaky gut').[223] This process has been linked to multiple diseases including dementia, cancer and diabetes.[224,225]

This information has been widely reported on blogs and anti-gluten websites across the globe which are keen to spread their message. Many fans of his research have used it to support their vision of a completely 'Gluten Free' world but, contrary to popular belief, this is not what he actually supports! Gluten- and grain-free diets are massively on trend, but before we rush to our store cupboards and furiously empty out all gluten-containing products, let's get some perspective. I want to put forward a few alternative arguments as to why gluten-free lifestyles may have worked for some people before we stamp traditional sourdough with a biohazard warning.

• Is it us or gluten? There are a lot of poor-quality products that contain gluten, such as breads, cereals and pasta (to name a few), and these ingredients form a major part of our diets. It's no wonder we are getting sick. Cereals for breakfast, 'healthy' tuna sandwich for lunch, pasta salad for dinner … sound familiar? We are barraging our bodies with quick-releasing sugars and what's more disturbing is the influx of 'gluten-free' products that are just as unhealthy as the original. Before going gluten free, ask yourself: what else is in your diet? A gluten-free version is not necessarily a healthier alternative and it bears all the hallmarks of the 'low-fat' movement. We all know where that has led us!

• Is it your gut bugs or gluten? The incidence of Coeliac Disease doubling every 15 years perhaps relates to shifts in our microbiome (among many other factors).[226] Changes in our gut bacteria population may be the underlying cause of symptoms that people are experiencing,[226] not necessarily just gluten. When patients remove gluten-containing products from their diet in place of whole foods and quality sources of complex carbohydrate (like lentils and sweet potato) they may have shifted their microbe population for the better. Their resolution of symptoms may be because of an improved microbe population or more conscientious food choices rather than a sensitivity to gluten. As we become more proficient at monitoring microbiome patterns and how the microbiome changes, further research will herald more interesting hypotheses in this field.

• It's more complicated than we think. It's very reductionist and unscientific to simply blame gluten for everything wrong with us. Like most things in nutrition and human physiology, the story goes deeper. Food has multiple interactions with our bodies. Instead of scapegoating a single protein in bread (a food that's been a staple for centuries and responsible in part for the quick expansion of the human race), I think we should turn our attention to the addition of phytochemical-rich foods and lack thereof in modern diets.

It's very reductionist and unscientific to simply blame gluten for everything wrong with us.

We all need to pack more nutrition into our diets. I know that essential micronutrients, fibre, proteins and fat are what our bodies are yearning for, so beige, gluten-containing foods don't make a daily appearance on my plate. Instead of filling up with poor-quality breads and pastas alone, give your body the full complement of nutrition and you'll be surprised at its self-healing ability.

If you do recognise an issue with gluten, keep a food diary and speak to your doctor or a nutrition practitioner. There are many ways to get good-quality carbohydrate and fibre onto our plates without consuming gluten. If you do, with the support of a practitioner, choose to remove gluten-containing products from your diet, my favourite foods to take their place include pulses and legumes, sweet potato, quinoa, whole rice and bean pastas.

I realise I may come under fire for not actively discouraging a gluten-free lifestyle and giving options for those who want to go gluten free, especially since the current evidence seems to suggest the majority of us do not have a problem with gluten-containing products, but here's my rationale.

Protecting a patient from the barrage of medical testing that comes with investigating the cause of symptoms like pain and abdominal bloating is a win. Time and time again I see patients (in many cases young women) being bounced from colonoscopy to ultrasound, to hysteroscopy, to blood test to biopsy. If the simple elimination of a food for a short period of time leads to improvement of sometimes debilitating symptoms, why obstruct it? I'd like to think that we are open-minded enough to appreciate the rationality of being completely wrong about our perceptions of gluten in the future. The jury is still out on it, but for now I don't encourage gluten-free lifestyles without due reason.

Supplements

Strolling into a speciality health-food and supplement store for the first time is quite an overwhelming experience, with so many ingredient options.

It's a bit like attending a raw vegan meet and greet; you're interested and it seems lovely, but you know you don't belong. Trust me, we've all been there. Rest assured, just like in conventional supermarkets, the majority of products available are well-branded garbage.

How do you know which supplement is good quality? Which probiotic is the best? Do I need this brown rice protein powder? Unfortunately, with 'health' products, the variability in quality of content is, well … varied. These aren't pharmaceutical products and as such are not held to the same standards. This, among other reasons, is why I'm a fan of getting your nutrition straight from the source: whole foods!

The best supplement for your body is a wide variety of food with nothing added. You can get the majority of minerals, vitamins, macronutrients and much more from a wholefoods diet, focused around colourful vegetables.[227] But, if you do feel you need to use a supplement, please do so under the guidance of a physician, registered nutritionist or dietician. Just because these tablets are available over the counter does not guarantee their safety.[228]

As you can tell, I'm really sceptical about overuse of supplementation. Despite our best efforts, we still have little understanding of human physiology. A reductionist approach to replacing micronutrients in isolation using high-dose pills is a concept I have reservations about.

Our public health history is dotted with medicine and supplement advice that we once thought was appropriate at a population level, but now we find ourselves backtracking on.[229,230] Our new knowledge of how highly individualised we are will soon overhaul our blanket one-size-fits-all approaches to both medicine and supplementation[231,232] and I'm excited about the future of tailored micronutrient regimens.

We already know that supplements can have either a detrimental or beneficial effect, depending on the person taking them. Factors like whether a patient smokes, what their general diet is like and if they already have precancerous lesions all impact the effect of these widely available pills from the health stores.[230,233] Taking a random multi-vitamin every day has consistently been shown in large trials to not positively affect our health.[234,235] Even if it improves your vitamin levels on a blood test, the effect on mortality and morbidity has not been shown to be significant. We are more complicated than a collection of a few chemical compounds, so save your pounds for some real nutrients and spend it on good-quality whole food.[236]

Furthermore, studies that used isolated plant chemicals (e.g. resveratrol and curcumin) and had patients arbitrarily supplement with them at high doses did not find them beneficial.[237,153] This just goes to show that the context in which these chemicals are introduced to the body is very

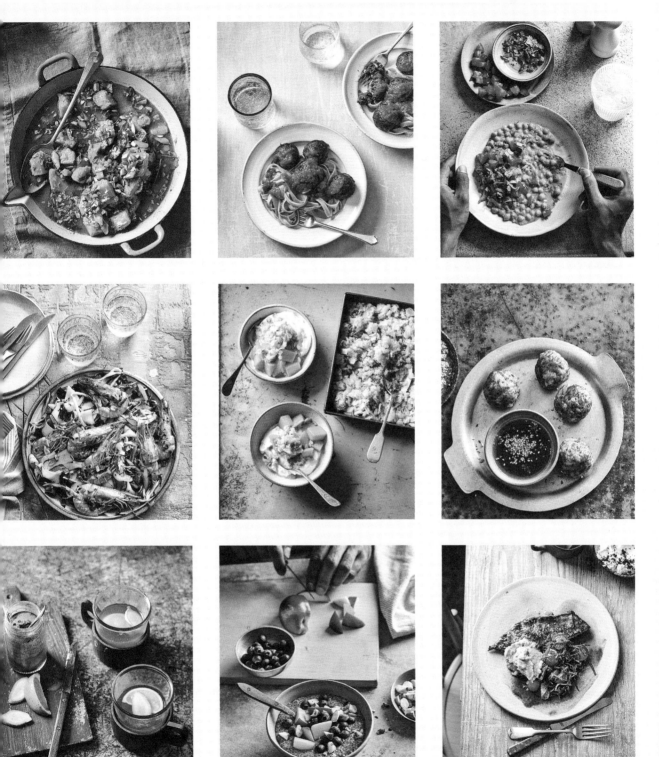

59 Introduction

important. The benefits of food are more than just a sum of compounds in different doses and I think it is naïve to think of supplementing in this way.

Having said all this, I do believe supplementation with certain micronutrients is worthwhile discussing with your practitioner, as a lot of people tend to be deficient in them, especially in the UK.

Vitamin D

This is essentially impossible to get from your diet. We create this vitamin via a reaction that happens in our skin on exposure to UV radiation, so levels tend to be low if you live in a part of the world that's often deprived of sunlight … like the British Isles. And this is a problem when we consider how important vitamin D is.

There is an industry trying to capitalise on your fear of being deficient, but I want to reassure you that you do not need to spend extortionate amounts of money to achieve a healthy life.

A master hormone, vitamin D is unique in its dual role as a regulator of genes and calcium balance. It's important in depression, bone health, cancer and the UK population is largely deficient, particularly Asian and African populations. It doesn't surprise me to see low vitamin D levels across many people in clinic and it is a standard test whenever I order bloods. Considering our ancestry and how our bodies are designed to function, it seems vitamin D has become a problem since we've stopped running around outside for the majority of our daylight hours.[238] There is controversy as to whether vitamin D levels are a marker of poor health or the cause of disease. On balance, my opinion is to have this level checked and there is enough evidence for me to believe it is worth supplementing.[239,240,241]

Vitamin B12

This is a must for all 100 per cent plant-based eaters[242] and something to consider for omnivores who only indulge in a steak every couple of weeks, like myself. Vitamin B12 is found in meat, fish and eggs and is a vital component of our diets. Anyone with fatigue, dementia or numbness sensation gets their vitamin B12 level checked in my clinic – it's standard practice.

Iron

Sources of iron include tofu, beans, lentils, nuts, seeds and – of course – dark leafy greens. But iron is a tricky subject. Its absorption varies from person to person and commonly we see deficiencies that are masked. Again, anyone with 'tired-all-the-time' symptoms gets their iron levels checked, alongside many other checks that are in a physician's differential diagnosis. I keep seeing iron supplement advertisements offering quick fixes for low energy levels. Fatigue is not solely caused by iron deficiency. Please see your doctor before you assume it is a low iron problem and start swigging back ferrous-sulphate drinks! In some cases, iron supplementation is necessary and it's worth discussing with your doctor the type of replacement that is suitable for you.

Omega-3 (EPA/DHA/algae source)

I think most people don't consume their oily fish quota for the week, and with new concerns arising from the mercury content in some fish species like sardines and anchovies I personally opt for an algae-based Omega-3 supplement (as well as eating other oily fish). Omega-3 is a vital fatty acid that we need for brain function, hormone production and cell membrane structure.[243]

There is some evidence for its cardioprotective role and this can explain why ingredients such as seaweed, extra-virgin olive oil and flaxseeds are heart healthy, but there is scepticism around these claims.[244,245] There's even an interesting suggestion that it has a role in depression,[246] behaviour[247] and traumatic brain injury recovery.[248] For now, I pop a pill every morning to keep myself in check, and my opinion is that a supplement with the long-chain Omega-3 fatty acids (called EPA and DHA) is worth it.

Nutraceuticals

There isn't strong enough evidence for me to recommend these for everyone, but nutraceuticals and whole food supplements are one to watch. They could potentially be a better alternative to synthetic vitamins when whole food convenience

is not an option. Some really interesting trials are looking at their effects on cancer[24] and diabetes, but for now, whole foods are where I recommend your daily micronutrients come from.

'First do no harm' is an oath we all take as medical professionals, and without a clear benefit or use for a supplement I recommend them with caution. I always tell patients that the best nutritional strategy is real food rather than fortified grains or cereals. And if you rely on fortified products to ensure you get your vitamins, you'd be better off just taking a pill to ensure the correct daily dosage.[249] Although the public health bodies have decided fortification of our food with vitamins is beneficial, I really don't think this is the most pragmatic, long-term approach. We need to educate not nanny, and this is where I think we should focus our efforts. It's how we can potentially lift ourselves out of an epidemic of chronic disease and bouts of nutritional deficiencies that are re-emerging due to poor lifestyle. You cannot supplement or fortify out of illness a population that isn't educated on the importance of nutrition.

As a rule of thumb, if the quantities in a supplement's ingredient list are radically different from what you'd find in nature, I'd only take them on the advice of a professional. There is an industry trying to capitalise on your fear of being deficient, but I want to reassure you that you do not need to spend extortionate amounts of money to achieve a healthy life.

The doctor's principles of eating + living well

Whether it's to nurture your microbiome, maximise your genetic potential or even improve your mental wellbeing, everything appears to boil down to some core principles.

You don't need to buy separate books or specific ingredients to take care of different aspects of your health. A holistic approach to your diet and lifestyle is what most of us need. I've done the hard work of reading through the literature examining plant compounds, the effect of vegetable-focused diets, gut health, nutrigenomics, micronutrients, sleep, meditation, inflammation and eating times. I gauge opinion from experts and I have experience of working on the healthcare frontline as both a general practitioner and emergency doctor. I appreciate the difficulties of why a healthy lifestyle doesn't always top the list of priorities on a working day.

It would be ideal if we all got nine hours of restful sleep every night, had perfect seasonal produce available at the touch of a button, a personal trainer to motivate us and freshly cooked meals prepared according to our nutritional needs. But my aim is to underline the most important aspects of lifestyle that I think are genuinely achievable in modern life and have the most impact on wellness. I've condensed these into core principles of eating and living well, which are realistic goals everyone can aim for. Importantly, there is real evidence behind my suggestions and I've refined the wealth of science available into easy, actionable points.

• **Eat colourful foods.** This goes without saying. Nutrient-dense food and micronutrients are lacking in our modern diets. Two different vegetables at every mealtime, as many different colours as possible and variation is key. Experiment with different foods throughout the seasons and learn to complement foods with spice – my recipes will show you how!

• **Focus on plant protein.** We do not need to rely on meat as a sole source of protein. In fact, our preoccupation with protein in general moves the attention away from micronutrient density which I believe should be our primary concern. Plant proteins offer the best of all worlds: nutrient density, phytochemicals and more than adequate quantities of both fibre and protein.

• **Don't forget fibre.** Fibre is key to longevity, gut microbe functioning and therefore general health. We lack fibre. Our ancestors would have consumed vast quantities, which I believe protect against diseases of modern living. It is fundamental to properly feed the population of bugs that live in our guts to help us stay healthy.

• **Don't fear fats.** They are vital for your body's physical and mental function. Use good-quality sources that I discuss on page 41 and enjoy their tasty health-promoting properties.

• **Define your hours of eating.** This practice of 'fasting' is very easy to implement in most people's working life. A fast every now and then would be ideal, but a general rule is not to eat late in the day. For now, use defined hours of eating as your rule of thumb: try to stick within a 10–11-hour window and eat at regular times each day.

• Remove refined food from your diet. Eat whole foods as much as possible. I don't want to scare you into never touching crisps or deep-fried chips, or enjoying delicate, fragrant white rice again. But, for most of what you choose to put in your body, whole food is the most health-promoting option.

• Sleep your way to health. Melatonin, the hormone produced during sleep, has a vital role in circadian rhythm. Get into the habit of respecting your body's need to sleep as you would respect its need to eat. Seven to eight hours is minimum for an adult.

• Electronic daily detox. Technology is both an advantage and disadvantage of modern living. Our over-stimulated minds are the price we pay for constant communication and convenience. Get into the habit of putting the phone and laptop away in the evenings at least two hours before bed and turning down the lights in your home. Your well-rested mind will thank you for it!

• Daily movement. You do not need to follow an intense daily exercise regimen. Variety, very much like food, is what your body will appreciate. Yoga, stretch, strength and endurance are great options.

• Mindfulness. Sitting in an uncomfortable, cross-legged position for hours at a time is not the only method of practising mindfulness. Ten minutes of active rest is all you need. It could be deep breathing, it could be listening to soothing sounds, it could be a gentle reminder to take

30 seconds before opening up another web browser. The effects aren't immediate, but it is a hack for longevity, reducing inflammation and thriving in a fast-paced world. I've done a gratitude exercise daily for years and it gives a real perspective into the beauty of life.

No matter how many bells and whistles you put on the research, fad diets, the opinions of researchers, experts and Eastern medicine practitioners, these are the core messages. If you want more information on how to live a healthier lifestyle, visit www.thedoctorskitchen.com.

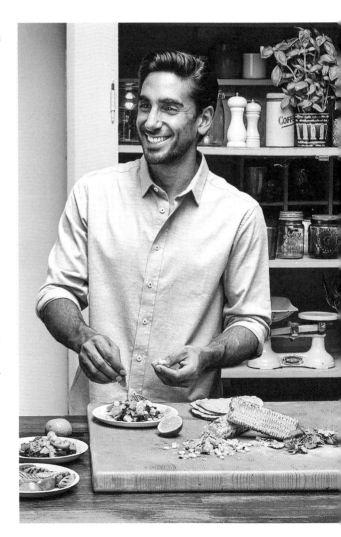

Introduction

Easy to start, simple to carry on

When I decided to start improving my diet and lifestyle, I needed to make my kitchen efficient.

Working late shifts, weekends and consecutive nights made it really difficult to pay attention to what I ate. I experimented with different kitchen appliances and gadgets in the hope that they'd speed up my progress on the journey to good health, but I soon realised I only needed a few kitchen staples and machines. I also developed some hacks that I'm sharing with you to keep you excited and confident in the kitchen. It'll ensure you don't fall into habits of relying on takeaway and convenience food that I used to depend on.

• **Tupperware is your friend.** Working in a busy A&E environment, odd shifts and hours mean I don't know where my next meal is coming from or when I can eat it. Tupperware and other airtight containers keep meals I've made in bulk fresh for my lunch the next day so I can avoid a trip to the dreaded hospital canteen!

• **Garlic, ginger, chilli.** These three ingredients form the flavour base of so many different cuisines including Italian, Chinese and Indian. They are always in my fridge door and are super-resistant to spoiling. Sometimes I grate them in bulk and put them in freezer bags. Supermarkets also sell them prepared and frozen. It's such a timesaver and you preserve a lot of the beneficial phytonutrients by preparing them this way.

• **Frozen food.** The reputation of frozen food has fluctuated in recent years but for busy families, frozen ingredients like peas, edamame and mixed vegetables are great to have to hand. If they've been frozen shortly after harvesting, these vegetables retain a lot of nutrition. Having peas in the freezer means you have super-quick access to a quality protein. I wouldn't depend on frozen vegetables on a daily basis, but as a reliable source of nutrition when you can't get to the shops after ten days on call, it's a convenient, healthy option.

• **Key kitchenware.** A quality ovenproof saucepan and frying pan, both with lids, are the two main cooking utensils in my kitchen. Other than that, all you need is a sharp knife, spice blender or coffee bean grinder, pestle and mortar, salad spinner, grater, mixing bowl, wooden chopping board and a vegetable peeler.

• **Cooking in bulk.** I have included a section in this book on cooking grains and pulses perfectly – see pages 94–100. Once you have a protein and a fibre-rich base, you can easily build fresh, nutrient-dense ingredients into your meals that taste completely new. Knowing I have some cooked puy lentils or chickpeas in the fridge means that dinner could be anything from an Italian-style stew to a Middle Eastern tagine.

• **Store-cupboard essentials.** I always have good-quality tinned foods in my cupboard (without added salt or sugar), such as adzuki beans, chickpeas, puy lentils or black beans. When you only have one vegetable in the fridge and it's late at night, having these fibre-rich staples to hand is brilliant for maintaining a healthy lifestyle.

• Dried legumes. Legumes are an underutilised source of nutrition that is cheap, easily available and a staple of the Mediterranean diet. I try to cook them from scratch (see page 94) and I have an extensive range of different types on my kitchen counter, from fava beans and black-eye peas to yellow split peas and beluga. I choose puy or yellow lentils when I'm in a rush, because they only take 30 minutes to cook from scratch.

• Nuts and seeds. These are high-quality whole sources of fat that are both satiating and healthy. My heart sinks when I have to re-educate patients about the use and nutritional benefits of nuts and seeds: a consequence of the 'low-fat' message is that there is genuine fear surrounding these bundles of nutrition. I buy them in bulk and keep them in airtight jars. Lightly roasted with a little honey and whole fruit or toasted in a dry frying pan with spices, they are delicious to snack on or use as meal toppers.

• Gadgets. There are so many culinary gadgets out there and I've tried most of them. My mother is obsessed with them and I think it has rubbed off on me! There are only two that I use regularly, however: a Nutribullet and a food processor. I use a Nutribullet for making everything from smoothies, my own nut milks, pastes and dressings and a food processor to make hummus, sauces and soups. But you can manage perfectly well without them.

• Spice shelf. Spices are your best friends in the kitchen. Give them the credit they deserve and allocate them their own drawer, cupboard or shelf. Invest in quality spices. It's far more economical to buy in bulk and keep them in airtight jars. If you use my recipes often enough, you'll soon get through them! My favourite prepared mixes include berbere, harissa, garam masala, dukkah, za'atar, ras el hanout and nasi goreng, and I make quite a few of these spice mixes myself (see pages 240–3). They'll transform anything from lightly steamed greens to your morning omelette.

• Pre-mixed spice pastes. They may not be as nutritious as fresh pastes, but they can be so useful when I come home from a late shift. Pastes will transform simple legumes into a curry from different cuisines. Add whatever else is left in the fridge and you have a much more nutrient-dense meal than a standard takeaway.

• Colours with every meal. One of the best 'hacks' I can give you is to look for the colour. With the new 'ten-a-day' guidelines I fear people are getting obsessed with having exactly the correct proportions of vegetables on their plates. If you have more than two coloured vegetables on your plate at each mealtime you're doing well. Add a couple of portions of fruit during the day and you're pretty much doing better than the entire country!

• Tips for when you fall off the wagon. Be mindful that it happens and enjoy it. Accept it then get back on track. Do not punish yourself for an indulgent weekend or festive season – these experiences shared with friends and family are what makes us human. The balance between a quality life and one that's restricted is very important. I never let my condition or the desire for a healthier lifestyle dictate the enjoyment of living and the memories I want to create.

Mindful cooking

For some people, cooking is not a relaxing or pleasurable activity. It is the last thing they want to do after a stressful day of work.

The anxiety of getting the right ingredients, chopping the vegetables correctly and avoiding ruining a meal is deeply unsettling.

Cooking is a constant learning process. Like any hobby, practice makes perfect and if you invest some effort into this life skill, the results are more than just pretty social-media pictures. I like to see the process of cooking as a type of mindfulness. A way of quietening the busy mind and concentrating on an activity to improve mental health.

I'm constantly learning new techniques and little hacks in the kitchen, but these suggestions are great if you're starting out and want to have a more relaxing time in the kitchen and improve your mood after a long day.

• Get into the right frame of mind. If you really don't feel like cooking and forcing it is going to make you feel anxious, then go easy on yourself and don't cook. Motivate yourself in the morning, or set a target the day before that you are going to cook a particular meal. The more you practise this, the more comfortable you get in the kitchen and the more likely it is that you'll have a positive experience.

• Have the essential ingredients for each recipe in your cupboards and fridge. Make sure you know where to get the ingredients locally, or have them already in your fridge. It makes the process

a lot smoother. Having the right spices and utensils that I have listed (see pages 64–5) will help to ensure you have all the necessities to cook well, all the time. Also, don't go shopping hungry!

• Play music. I find listening to music so important when cooking. It adds an extra element of comfort to the kitchen environment and I even have a particular playlist I cook to. Try creating your own list of songs that you really love – it'll keep you cooking!

• Mise en place. This is the art of preparing all your ingredients in the right quantities before you start. The reason TV chefs look so calm and collected on air is because everything is pre-washed, chopped and ready to cook with. Get into the habit of doing this before you turn the oven on or put the pan on the hob and you're less likely to burn your food or – even worse – cause an injury. I don't want to see any more kitchen-related accidents in A&E, please.

• Clean as you cook. There is nothing worse than coming back into a messy kitchen after enjoying a lovely meal and having to tidy up, and it's one of the many reasons we don't cook as often as we should. If you get into good habits it becomes effortless.

• Join forces. Just like having a personal trainer or a gym buddy, sometimes teaming up with a friend to make a meal is all the encouragement you need to start cooking. You can bounce ideas off each other, experiment and – importantly – you'll have someone to help with the chopping.

• Get the family in the kitchen. Bringing the family together during meal preparation is so helpful for children's development and the connection between food and health. All my vivid childhood memories are centred around that all-important place in the house. One of the best sessions I ran at the community kitchen I work at (Made in Hackney) was when we organised a parent-and-child cooking class. The kids were taught how to prepare fruit and make a smoothie while I showed the parents the benefits of cooking from a health point of view.

I really hope these suggestions make cooking a much easier and more pleasurable experience for you. After years of trial and error, these tips have really helped me to become more relaxed and proficient at the hob. Experiment, expect mistakes, but always enjoy the process.

I like to see the process of cooking as a type of mindfulness. A way of quietening the busy mind to improve mental health.

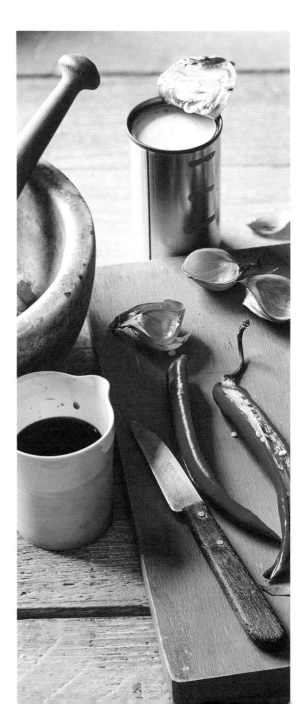

Introduction

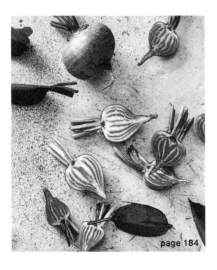

page 184

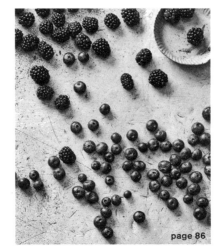

page 86

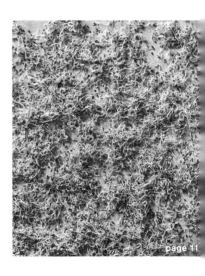

page 11

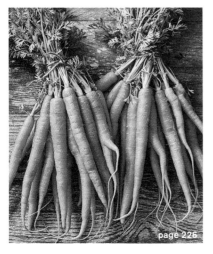

page 226

The Doctor's Favourites

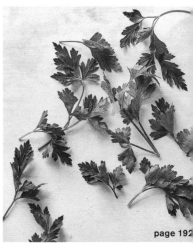

page 192

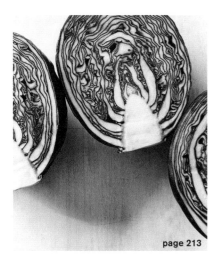

page 213

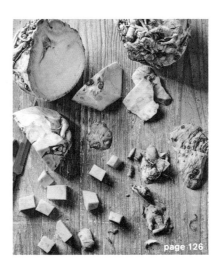

page 126

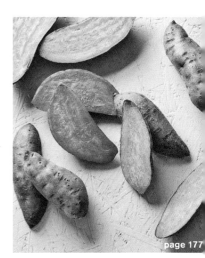

page 177

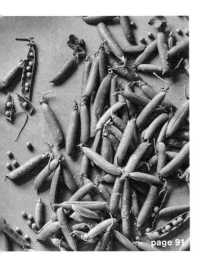
page 91

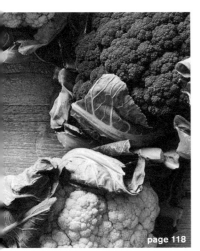
page 118

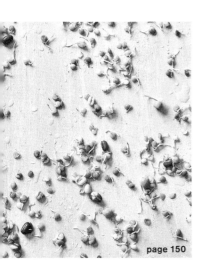
page 150

I've scattered features on my 'Doctor's Favourites' ingredients throughout the book. The aim of these is to give you a sense of how everyday ingredients are packed full of nutrients that have positive effects on our health. I hope they will inspire you to reconsider the power of the vegetables that line our supermarket shelves. They are far from mundane and are key to longevity and wellness.

What the doctor ordered

The aim of this cookbook is to take you on a journey of discovery and tell you why food is so important.

Food affects our cell structure, our population of microbes, our brain chemistry, even our genetic material. I want everybody, medical professionals included, to appreciate and recognise that…

> Plates are as powerful as Pills and Food is truly Medicine.

I hope this book empowers you to get more nutrient-dense foods onto your plates. By using a multitude of ingredients that are health promoting, I hope to show you that a healthy way of life is not mundane, bland or difficult. It's an enjoyable way of living that will transform your perspective and your health.

> By using a multitude of ingredients that are health promoting, I hope to show you that a healthy way of life is not mundane, bland or difficult.

We need to go back to basics. This book is the first step toward using diet in self care. Our minds and bodies can only achieve their full potential if given the right nutrition and environment. Food is the important conversation-starter about lifestyle medicine in modern healthcare. We are beautiful machines with intricate chemistry and the food we eat is just as complex.

Don't expect to find dishes in this book that promise to reverse cholesterol and 'clean out' clogged arteries. This is not a source of cure-all recipes. The exact proportions of macronutrients, specific ingredients and supplementation to help with health conditions are very individual and dependent on the patient and the cause. It's extremely naïve to think a one-size-fits-all approach works for everything. No book can deliver this promise to every reader. Each recipe in my book is likely to have a blood-sugar-stabilising effect, plenty of micronutrients, antioxidants and the ability to reduce inflammation, but it can't guarantee improvement – let alone reversal – of medical conditions. We are unique.

The principles of healthy living are what's important. Stick to these and you have the blueprint of a healthy life that allows you to reach your full potential.

Flavour and function are woven throughout all of my dishes which celebrate the beauty of food and its complex effects on the human body while also exciting your taste buds. Use these recipes as inspiration for how to get nutrient-dense, delicious and accessible food back into your diet. Get into the kitchen and explore – I want this book to be covered in spices, random ingredients and spills. It's what the doctor ordered.

The recipes

I've created 100 beautiful and easy recipes to slot into anyone's life. I have united the research with delicious foods. Everything from the choice of ingredients and the methods of cooking to the combination of spices has been influenced by the studies and the clinical research available. I truly hope you enjoy making them and sharing them with your loved ones. A meal is not just an opportunity to refuel or a collection of molecules that we need consume to sustain life. It is so much more than just this. It is medicine in the true sense of the word: a complex array of elements that have vast effects on our behaviour and life experiences. It is as complex and diverse as the universe itself and a perfect entry point to lifestyle medicine.

Recipe highlights

I've highlighted some recipes to get people interested in how food can have a role in helping prevent and manage certain conditions. But please remember, do not treat food as a pill; we shouldn't consider nutrition in isolation. Our entire lifestyle – that includes our sleep patterns, our stress and activity levels – has a role in helping us live healthier, happier lives.

These dishes are particularly colourful and contain a great selection of Omega-3 fats. They are full of whole ingredients that may prevent high blood pressure and issues with high cholesterol.

Meals with plenty of fibre, reduced sugar and refined carbohydrates, plus a variety of different vegetables is key to controlling blood sugar levels. I've highlighted those recipes that tick all these boxes.

These gut healthy recipes use a selection of different ingredients that may be beneficial for the functioning of our gut microbiome. They contain lots of different types of fibre, plenty of colour and a good dose of spice.

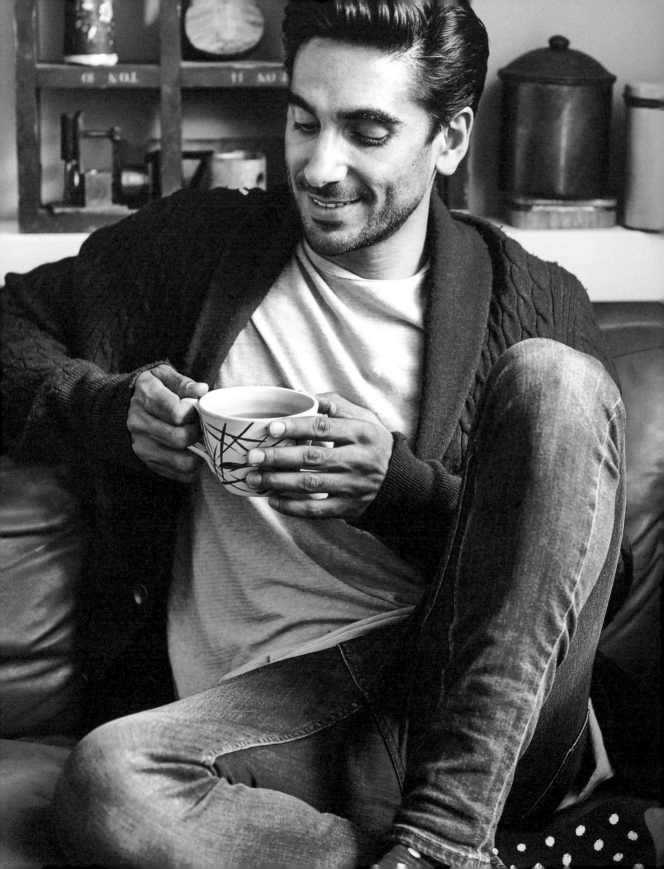

Breakfast

Before clinic, I must have something wholesome to eat. Without a decent breakfast that includes good-quality fats, fibre and protein I know the rest of the day is going to be hard work, but I try to ease myself gently into the first meal. I get up early, drink water, stretch or exercise and I like to prepare breakfast from scratch. In Indian cuisine, as well as many others, the first meal of the day is often a savoury one and working night shifts and odd hours, I've got used to breakfast not always being sweet. Every dish is a beautiful collection of micronutrient-dense ingredients, fibre, fats and protein: a perfect start to fuel your day and feel fantastic.

I love starting my day with this great mixture of greens. I created the dish around Christmas time using up the leftovers from a stuffing recipe and I now use cooked chestnuts in my recipes all the time. Their soft texture contrasts well with the firm broccoli, and the subtle thyme brings everything together. Broccoli stalks are packed with fibre that your gut microbes will thrive on, not to mention a concentrated source of phytochemicals. Be sure to use these delicious sources of nutrition.

Chestnut and Thyme Peas with Broccoli

serves 1

2 tbsp extra-virgin olive oil

100g broccoli, florets finely sliced and stalk trimmed and cubed

1 garlic clove, finely chopped

leaves from 4 thyme sprigs

50g peas (fresh or thawed)

50g cooked chestnuts

pinch of cayenne pepper

small knob of butter

1 egg

sea salt and freshly ground black pepper

Preheat the grill to medium.

Heat the oil in a large frying pan, add the cubed broccoli stalk and garlic and sauté for 3–4 minutes until lightly browned. Add the thyme leaves, broccoli florets and peas, crumble in the cooked chestnuts and add the cayenne pepper. Cover and cook for 2 minutes.

Meanwhile, melt the butter in a separate small frying pan over a medium heat, crack in the egg and fry for 1 minute, or until the white is cooked. Transfer the pan to the preheated grill and cook for 2–3 minutes, until the egg white is cooked but the yolk is still runny.

Serve the chestnuts and broccoli with the fried egg on top and season lightly with salt and pepper.

TIPS
+ Try making this with different vegetables such as cauliflower, asparagus or even chicory.
+ Swap the cayenne pepper for a different spice, such as dried chilli flakes or chipotle chilli, if you prefer.

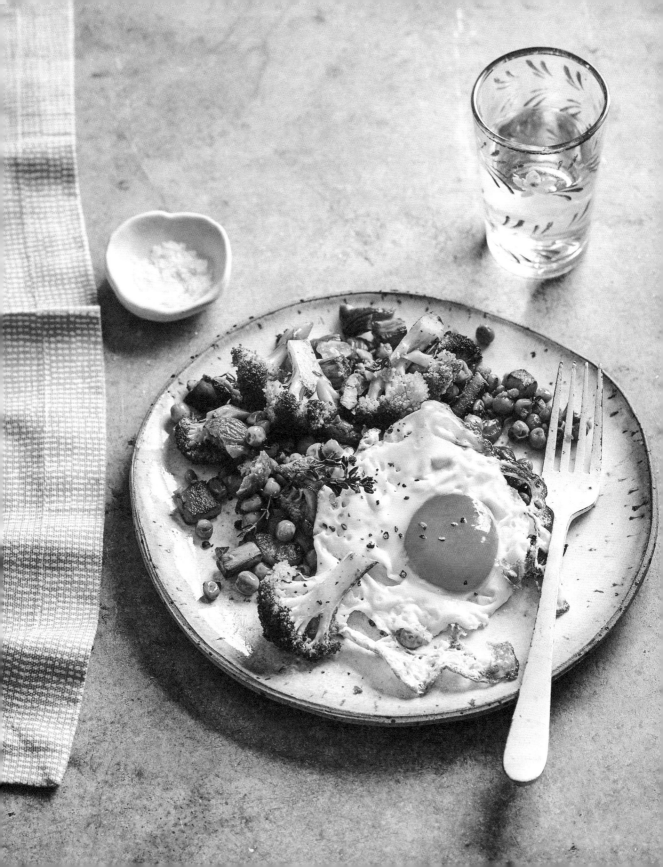

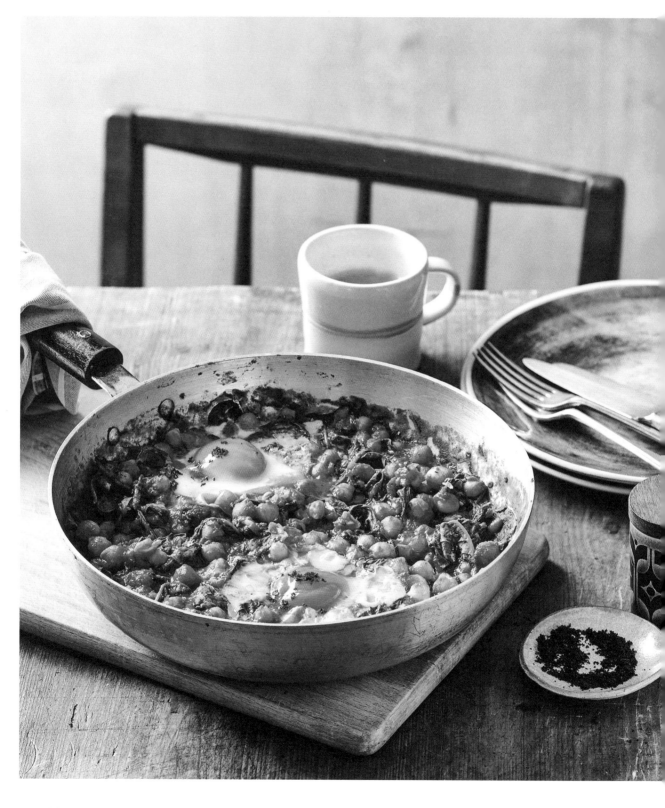

Breakfast

Sometimes there's nothing more delicious and satisfying than eggs in a spiced tomato sauce, with lashings of olive oil and tangy sumac. It's so easy to make and I've heightened the nutritional value of this classic dish by adding spinach and chickpeas to the tomatoes. Sumac is a potent antioxidant spice and gives the dish a refreshing, citrusy edge.

Spicy Baked Eggs with Tomatoes and Chickpeas

serves 2

3 tbsp extra-virgin olive oil

2 garlic cloves, finely chopped

leaves from 2 thyme sprigs

200g tinned chickpeas, drained and rinsed

2 tsp harissa paste

100g spinach leaves

200g passata or tinned chopped tomatoes

1 tsp dried chilli flakes

2 eggs

1 tsp sumac

sea salt and freshly ground black pepper

Preheat the grill to medium.

Heat 2 tablespoons of the olive oil in a large ovenproof frying pan, add the garlic and thyme leaves and sauté for 2 minutes, until the garlic has softened but not burnt.

Add the chickpeas and harissa paste and sauté for a further 2 minutes, then stir in the spinach, passata or chopped tomatoes and chilli flakes and bring to a simmer. When the mixture starts to simmer, carefully crack the eggs over it so they sit neatly on top.

Simmer for 2 minutes, then transfer the pan to the preheated grill and cook for 2–3 minutes, until the egg whites are cooked but the yolks are still runny (keep an eye on it to make sure the eggs don't overcook).

Remove from the grill, drizzle with the remaining olive oil, sprinkle with the sumac and season with salt and pepper.

Breakfast

The sheer depth of colour in this dish screams richness of nutrients. Cacao and blueberries are two of my favourite ingredients that pair perfectly in both flavour and positive effects on heart health. The ease with which this can be made means it's often something I put together in a rush before running to clinic. Its bitter-sweet flavour will energise the taste buds and the rich chemicals in the berries may protect from cognitive problems related to ageing.

Elegant Flavanol Porridge

serves 1

75g porridge oats

50g ground flaxseeds

200ml almond milk (or any nut milk), plus extra if needed

1 tsp ground cinnamon

2 tsp cacao powder

2 tbsp honey

100g blueberries (or blackberries)

20g black sesame seeds, toasted

Toast the oats and ground flaxseeds in a dry saucepan over a medium heat for 2 minutes, stirring frequently, until aromatic.

Pour the milk into the pan and stir, then add the cinnamon, cacao powder and half the honey and simmer for 4–5 minutes, stirring, until thickened, adding extra milk or water to loosen it if needed. Remove from the heat.

Heat the berries in a small frying pan with a splash of water until their skins split and they infuse the water with their colour, then add the remaining honey to thicken.

Serve the porridge warm, topped with the berries and sprinkled with the toasted sesame seeds.

A slice of this fibre-rich nut roast will keep me going until lunch. I usually make it on a Sunday and eat it throughout the week, lightly toasted and served up for breakfast with different twists each day. Sometimes I have it with a fried egg on top or occasionally, with a dollop of delicious probiotic yoghurt with some tahini, parsley and chilli folded through it. We need to challenge the concept that our first meal should be a refined carbohydrate-rich meal lacking in nutrients – hopefully this will keep you out of the cereal aisle! Caraway seeds give it a characteristic rye-bread flavour and help ease the digestion of the pulses.

Breakfast Nut Roast

serves 4

200g cashews, soaked in water for 30 minutes, drained and rinsed

200g cooked chestnuts

2 tsp extra-virgin olive oil, plus extra for greasing

1 tsp caraway seeds

1 red onion, finely diced

needles from 2 rosemary sprigs, chopped

200g red lentils, soaked in water for 30 minutes, drained and rinsed

50g sun-dried tomatoes in oil, drained and chopped

200ml water

sea salt and freshly ground black pepper

Preheat the oven to 200°C/180°C fan/gas 6 and grease a roughly 6 x 16cm (about 6cm-deep) loaf tin with oil.

Put the cashews and chestnuts in a food processor and pulse until you have a roughly ground mixture. Transfer to a bowl.

Heat the oil in a large frying pan over a medium heat add the caraway seeds, onion and rosemary and sauté for a few minutes until soft. Add the lentils, sun-dried tomatoes and water, bring to a simmer and cook for 20 minutes, until the lentils are soft and mushy.

Add the lentils to the nut mixture in the bowl, season with salt and pepper and mix to combine. The mixture will be stodgy and should hold together. If it is too dry, add a splash of water.

Tip the mixture into the greased baking tin, press it down and level it out and bake in the oven for 45–50 minutes until the top is browned. Remove from the oven and allow to cool before removing from the tin.

Keep the nut roast in the fridge for up to a week, slicing off a chunk when you need a filling protein- and fibre-rich herby snack!

+ TIP
Feel free to experiment with the spices. Try replacing caraway seeds with fennel or cumin.

Oats are one of the easiest ways to introduce fibre into our diets and I usually have them a couple of times a week. It's also a good opportunity to use fresh fruit, a mixture of nuts and some unusual spices to give you a kick-start. I tend to grate whatever fruit I have available into my porridge as I cook it, but try experimenting with carrots. They are a rich source of fibre and full of antioxidants like beta-carotene, but their benefits may go even further (see page 226).

serves 1

Ginger and Carrot Oats

60g porridge oats

15g sunflower seeds

15g flaked almonds, plus
    extra to serve

150ml almond milk (or dairy milk),
    plus extra if needed

1 pear, grated (about 50g), plus
    extra slices to serve (optional)

1 carrot, grated (about 30g)

1 tsp freshly grated root ginger

1 tsp ground cinnamon, plus
    extra to serve

1 tsp honey

Toast the oats, seeds and almonds in a dry saucepan over a medium heat for a couple of minutes, stirring frequently, until lightly browned.

Pour the milk into the pan and stir, then add the rest of the ingredients and simmer for 2–3 minutes, stirring, until thickened, adding extra milk to loosen it if needed.

Serve the oats warm with an extra sprinkle of cinnamon, flaked almonds and some extra sliced pear if you wish.

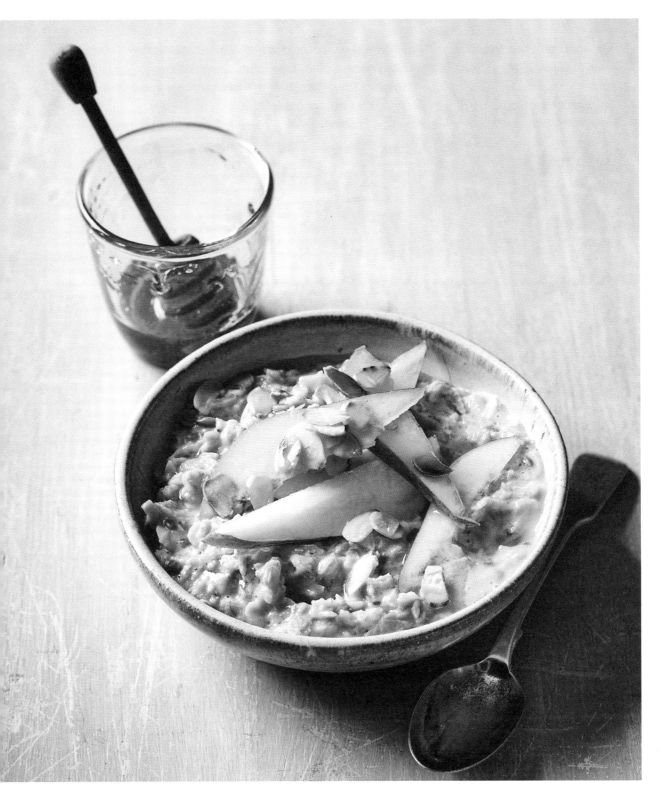

A simple omelette with a few extra ingredients blended into it can be the most satisfying and nutritious meal. I'm always keen to use lentils in dishes because they are a great source of fibre: a macronutrient that is lacking in a lot of our diets and is vital for health. A couple of servings of lentils pretty much covers your required intake for the day. This quick dish is much more satisfying than a smoothie and has tons of micronutrients. If you have one, a bullet blender aerates the mixture, giving it a fluffy, light texture when cooked, but you can use a food processor.

Garam Lentil Omelette

serves 1

2 tbsp cooked puy lentils
    (from a packet if you like)

small handful of spinach (about 20g)

2 eggs

2 tbsp extra-virgin olive oil

½ tsp dried chilli flakes, plus extra
    to serve (optional)

3–4 coriander stalks,
    roughly chopped

½ tsp garam masala (see page 240
    for my own blend)

small handful of rocket (about 15g)

sea salt and freshly ground
    black pepper

Preheat the grill to medium.

Put the lentils, spinach, eggs, 1 tablespoon of the oil, the chilli flakes, coriander and garam masala in a blender or food processor with a pinch each of salt and pepper and blend until smooth.

Heat the rest of the oil in a non-stick frying pan. Pour in the mixture from the blender and cook over a medium heat for about 2 minutes, until the bottom of the omelette is set. Transfer the pan to the preheated grill for 2–3 minutes until the top of the omelette is cooked.

Serve the omelette with the rocket and a sprinkle of chilli flakes (if you wish).

TIPS
+ If you have more time, make an aloo gobi (see my Colourful Gobi on page 156) to serve with this, and you have a satisfying, colourful Indian-inspired brunch!
+ Experiment with different spices: try harissa paste or even Jerk Paste (see page 249) instead of chilli and garam masala if you're feeling brave.

I have a lot of fun in the kitchen making fusion dishes of classic British breakfasts and brunch fare. My friends absolutely love this easy twist on beans with scrambled eggs and I'm sure you will, too. The spices and herbs cut through the heaviness of the beans and the fresh tomato with white onion 'crunch' delivers a burst of flavour. Black beans are a mighty protein source for people with a largely plant-based diet and the eggs are a much-needed source of vitamin B12 for those who eat a vegetarian diet.

Spicy Scrambled Eggs
with Curried Beans

serves 2

1 tbsp coconut oil

1 tsp freshly grated root ginger

1 tsp cumin seeds

½ tsp dried chilli flakes

1 spring onion (or ¼ white onion) finely chopped

4 eggs, beaten

25g cherry tomatoes, quartered

sea salt

For the curried beans

1 tbsp coconut oil

½ white onion, finely diced, plus extra to serve

½ tsp freshly ground black pepper

½ tsp turmeric

½ tsp chilli powder

200g tinned black beans, drained and rinsed (or 100g dried black beans, cooked 'perfectly' – see page 97)

50g spring greens, finely chopped

10g coriander, leaves and stalks finely chopped, plus extra leaves to serve

100g tinned chopped tomatoes

To make the curried beans, melt the coconut oil in a saucepan over a medium heat, add the onion, black pepper, turmeric, chilli powder and a pinch of salt and sauté for 2 minutes until the onion has softened but not browned.

Add the black beans, spring greens and coriander and cook, stirring, for 1 minute, then tip in the chopped tomatoes, bring to a simmer and cook for 2 minutes. Cover and remove from the heat.

To cook the eggs, heat the coconut oil in a frying pan, add the ginger, cumin and chilli, season with a pinch of salt and sauté for 1 minute. Add the spring onion and fry for a further 1–2 minutes, then pour in the eggs and vigorously scramble with a wooden spoon until softly set.

Serve the beans with the eggs, topped with a pinch of diced white onion and the cherry tomatoes for texture, and a scattering of coriander leaves.

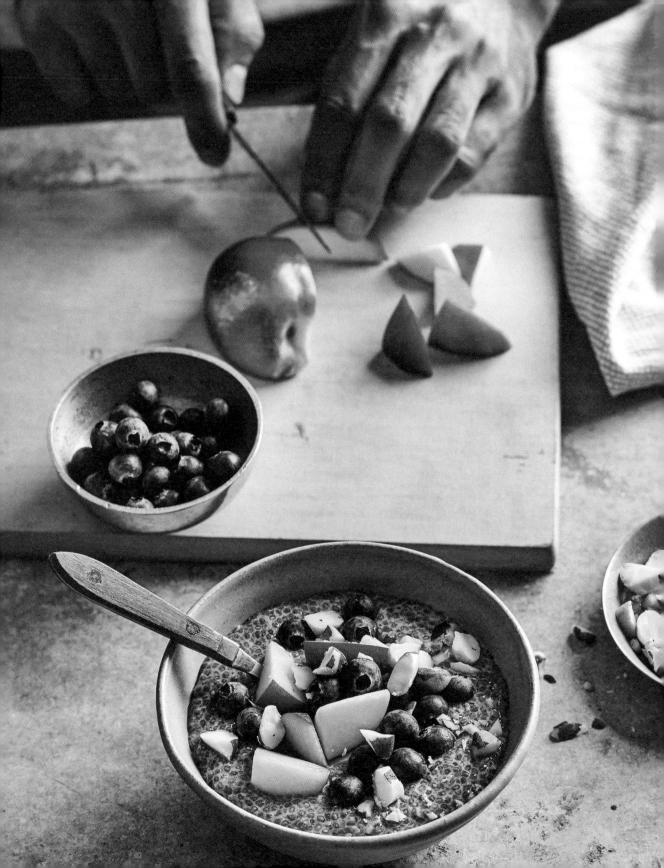

When I'm working in A&E and I need to be out of the door by 6am, I don't have time to create a lovely Instagram-worthy poached egg with miso quinoa. I need something nourishing and ready to chow down straight away. Preparing breakfast the night before is a huge bonus: it makes your morning much less stressful, and an essential-fat-rich seed like chia fuels you until lunch. Eating these gelatinous pods reminds me of a sweet Indian drink, akin to a sundae, called 'falooda', that I drank as a child. However, those are made with sickly sweet rose syrup and this is far better for you!

Overnight Cardamom and Chia Breakfast

serves 1

2 tbsp chia seeds

180ml almond milk
  (or dairy/coconut milk)

½ tsp ground cinnamon

½ tsp freshly grated root ginger

seeds from 3 green cardamom pods

1 tsp honey

Toppings

crushed nuts of your choice

frozen berries, or slices of
  orange or nectarine (or whatever
  fruit is in season)

Combine all the ingredients in a bowl, stir, cover and place in the fridge overnight.

Serve the cardamom and chia mixture straight from the fridge the next morning, garnished with crushed nuts and/or berries.

TIP
+ I find 10g chia seeds to 60ml fluid is the perfect ratio for me, but feel free to change the quantities as you like.

ALTERNATIVES: CRANBERRIES   BLACKCURRANTS
                  CHERRIES   RASPBERRIES

DOCTOR'S
FAVOURITES

Blueberries and Blackberries

I always include berries in my weekly shopping basket because I enjoy their bitter-sweet taste and intense colour, and their concentration of phytochemicals potentially reduces the risk of dementia and heart disease. Fresh berries can be expensive out of season, but frozen varieties are just as nutrient-dense and very convenient for cooking. I like to make an indulgent sweet berry sauce to pour over oats and nuts in the morning by throwing frozen berries into a saucepan with a splash of water and a touch of honey and cooking them down for a few minutes until soft. It is an easy way to get these plant chemicals into your system and the research shows that they are heat stable, too, so cooking them doesn't significantly reduce their nutritional qualities.

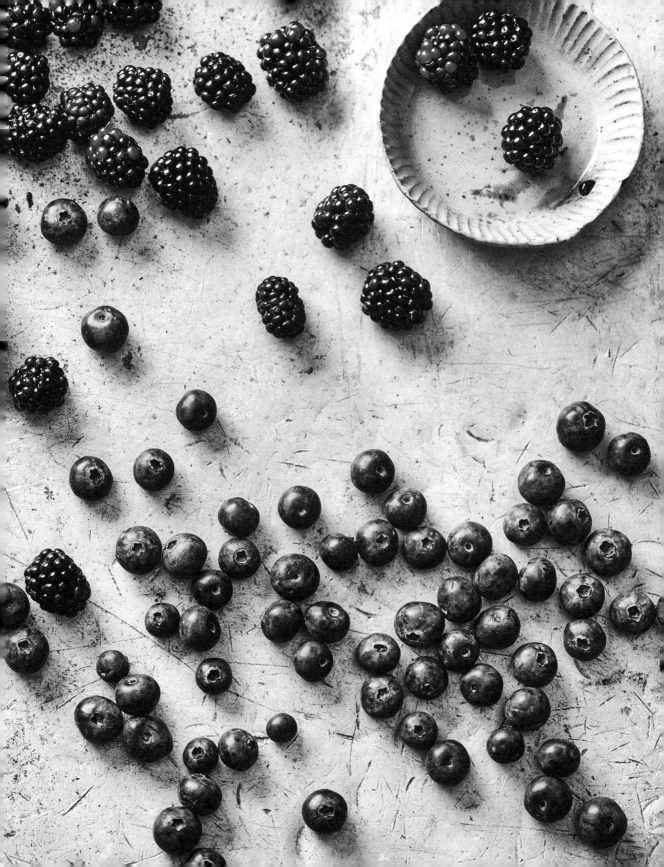

This breakfast transports me to my travels through the beautiful country of Jordan. I was at a medical conference in the UAE and decided to take a few days off, rent a car and drive down the Jordanian coastline. Before the journey I fuelled myself on a beautifully spiced platter of wholesome food. It inspired this dish and has become a favourite of mine ever since. Mackerel is a rich source of Omega-3 – an essential fat commonly lacking in our diets. Sumac is one of the world's richest sources of antioxidants. Its lemony tang makes it a staple spice in Middle Eastern dishes.

Middle Eastern Mackerel with Green Hummus

serves 2

---

3 tsp za'atar, plus extra to serve

3 tbsp extra-virgin olive oil, plus extra to serve

2 fresh mackerel (or sardine) fillets (about 100g each), skin on

100g cherry tomatoes, halved

50g baby spinach leaves, finely shredded

1 tsp sumac

2 tbsp labneh (or full-fat probiotic yoghurt)

sea salt and freshly ground black pepper

For the green hummus

400g tin chickpeas, drained and rinsed (or 200g dried chickpeas, cooked 'perfectly' – see page 96)

75g garden peas (fresh or thawed)

1 garlic clove

pinch of sea salt

½ tsp dried chilli flakes

1 tsp ground cumin

2 tbsp extra-virgin olive oil (or cold-pressed oil of your choice)

juice of ½ lemon

50ml cold water

Combine the za'atar with 1 tablespoon of the oil and smother the mackerel fillets in the za'atar oil. Place the fillets skin-side down on a grill pan on medium heat and cook for 2 minutes, then flip them over and cook for a further minute. Remove and set aside.

To make the green hummus, put all the ingredients in a food processor or blender and blitz until smooth.

Toss the tomatoes and spinach leaves in a bowl with the rest of the oil, the sumac and a sprinkling of salt and pepper.

Serve the grilled mackerel fillets with the tomato and spinach salad, the labneh, sprinkled with a dusting of za'atar and drizzled with oil, and the hummus.

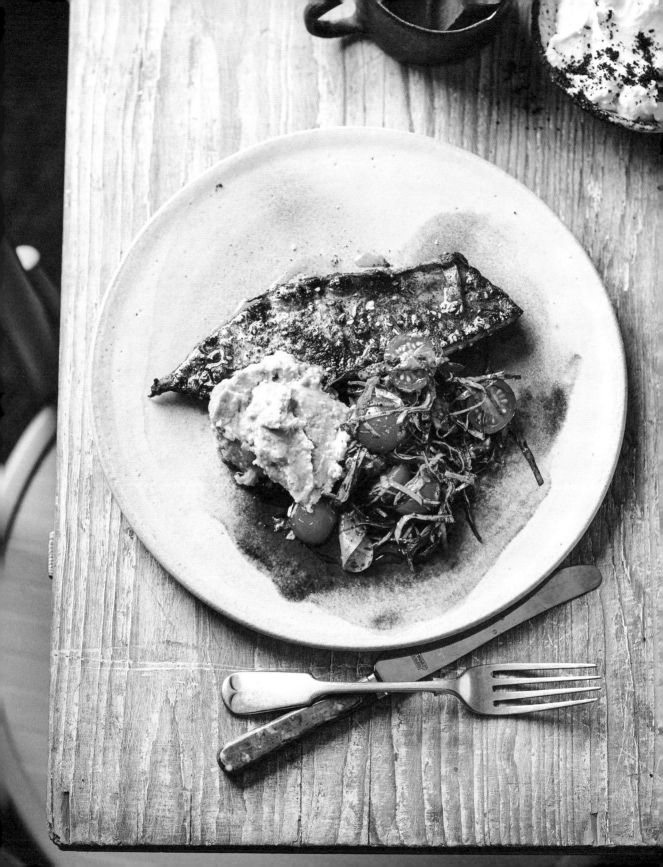

If I find carrots and peas in my kitchen, I know breakfast is sorted. Better still, if there's potato or another starchy vegetable to hand, we're definitely in business. Subji is a staple breakfast or brunch dish in my house. Full of flavour, colour and gorgeous ingredients, you'll never look at 'boring' carrots and peas in the same way again. Adding a bit of heat and spice creates a truly delicious and exceptionally quick meal.

Carrot and Pea Subji with Coriander Yoghurt

serves 2

2 tbsp coconut oil, butter or ghee

2 tsp black mustard seeds

1 tsp garam masala (see page 240 for my own blend)

3cm piece of root ginger, peeled and grated

3 carrots, cut into 1cm cubes

150g frozen peas

sea salt and freshly ground black pepper

For the coriander yoghurt

50g natural yoghurt

small bunch of coriander, finely chopped

½ tsp chilli powder

Melt the coconut oil, butter or ghee in a frying pan and add the mustard seeds. When the mustard seeds start to release their aroma and crackle, add the garam masala, seasoning and grated ginger, along with the carrots.

Cook gently for 3–4 minutes until the carrots are soft, then toss in the peas, cover with a lid, and cook for 1 minute. Remove from the heat and set aside.

Mix the yoghurt, coriander and chilli powder in a bowl and serve with the vegetables and a small portion of brown rice or a fresh wholemeal Indian bread, if you like.

TIP

+ You could add finely diced sweet potato to the carrots, but you may need to cook it for a further 4 minutes until softened, before adding the peas.

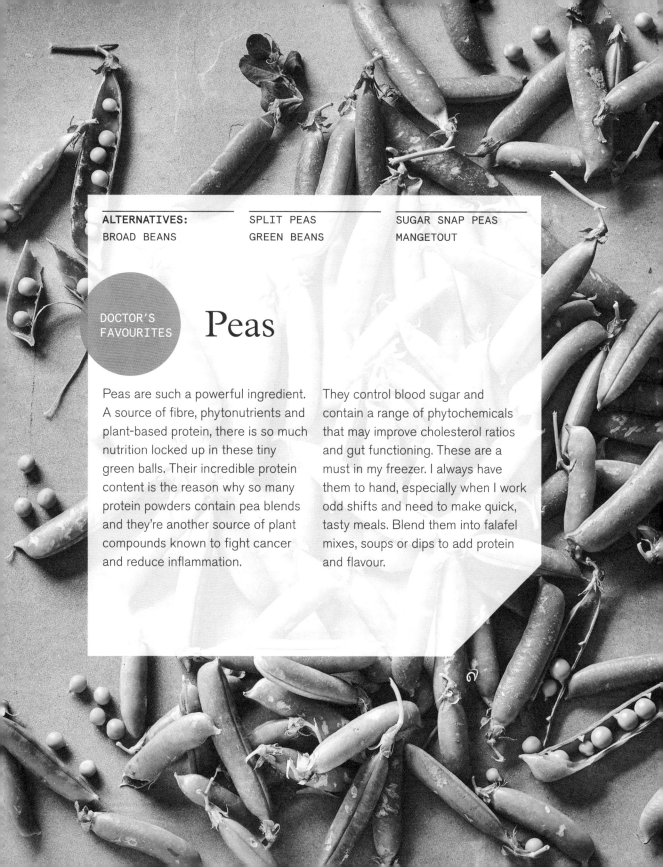

ALTERNATIVES:
BROAD BEANS

SPLIT PEAS
GREEN BEANS

SUGAR SNAP PEAS
MANGETOUT

DOCTOR'S
FAVOURITES

Peas

Peas are such a powerful ingredient. A source of fibre, phytonutrients and plant-based protein, there is so much nutrition locked up in these tiny green balls. Their incredible protein content is the reason why so many protein powders contain pea blends and they're another source of plant compounds known to fight cancer and reduce inflammation.

They control blood sugar and contain a range of phytochemicals that may improve cholesterol ratios and gut functioning. These are a must in my freezer. I always have them to hand, especially when I work odd shifts and need to make quick, tasty meals. Blend them into falafel mixes, soups or dips to add protein and flavour.

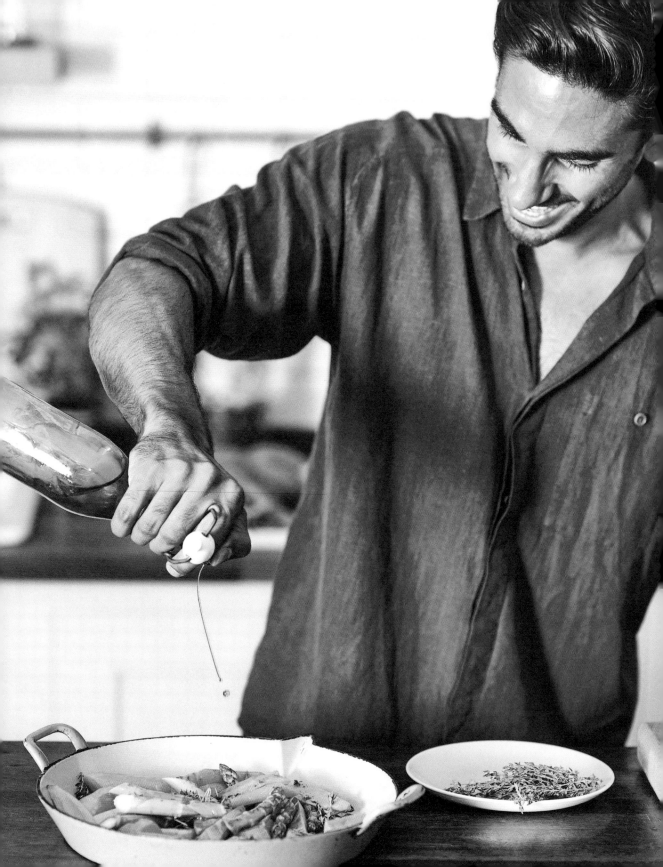

Sides and small plates

Sometimes, all I need to make a meal complete, satisfying and enjoyable is a small side dish made with simple, nutrient-dense ingredients. I've decided to dedicate the first part of this chapter to teaching you how to cook some key ingredients. I tend to cook rice, lentils and sweet potato in batches that keep in the fridge for 3–4 days. Then, all you need are a few extra fresh ingredients to transform these fibre-rich staples into something vibrant and tasty. This little hack is essential for juggling a busy work/life balance and keeping exciting yet quick-to-prepare meals on the menu at home. Learning how to cook these ingredients well is critical to creating nutritious dishes on a regular basis.

Perfect legumes

Legumes are one of the main elements of the Mediterranean diet, which has a strong influence on my cooking, and if you're a fan of my recipes on social media you'll notice how often I use them.

I always soak legumes. Always. Traditional cooking methods were instilled in me from childhood, when I remember seeing the kitchen worktop at home covered with big pans of water in which lentils, beans and pulses had been soaking overnight. Despite my busy schedule I still manage to do this often. By leaving the pan of water by the sink I don't forget about the soaking pulses. Also, when I was training as a general practitioner in Brighton, my housemates will testify that I used to sprout mung beans, chickpea and brown lentils on a weekly basis!

There is a scientific theory behind our ancestors' traditional technique for preparing legumes for cooking. Soaking lentils removes 'anti-nutrients' that are chemicals which bind to minerals. Without proper soaking, legumes can adversely affect the absorption of minerals like zinc and magnesium, plus the anti-nutrient chemicals themselves can irritate the gut lining. Even though a lot of books and chefs claim you can cook lentils straight from the packet, I wouldn't skip this important step. Different legumes require different soaking and cooking times, too.

Sprouting takes the soaking a step further to the point where you essentially 'germinate' the seed. By keeping it warm and damp, sprouts emerge from the pulses and you're left with a crunchy and satisfying ingredient. There are a number of benefits to sprouting, including improved protein availability, fewer anti-nutrients that can interfere with micronutrient absorption and potentially more fibre and antioxidants. Those unable to tolerate legumes may fare much better when they are sprouted, plus they are both delicious and versatile. Although they are now starting to appear in supermarkets, I've included a simple method for sprouting at home (see page 97).

I would like to point out that despite their unfortunate name, 'anti-nutrients' (also known by names such as phytates and tannins) have a very important role in human health. They're known to have an antioxidant effect, stabilise blood sugar and reduce inflammation. It could be another reason why we see health benefits in populations that include legumes as a staple in their diet, beyond simply the fact that they provide extra fibre. Just like medicines, anti-nutrients are likely to have a 'therapeutic window': too high a concentration of them causes problems, too few and you are unlikely to reap their benefits. Proper preparation of legumes vastly reduces the concentration of anti-nutrients so they are tolerable for consumption. In summary, please don't be afraid of legumes because of anti-nutrients. There appears to be a lot of scaremongering from people who claim they cause health problems: if you do notice a problem, please speak to your doctor or nutritionist about it.

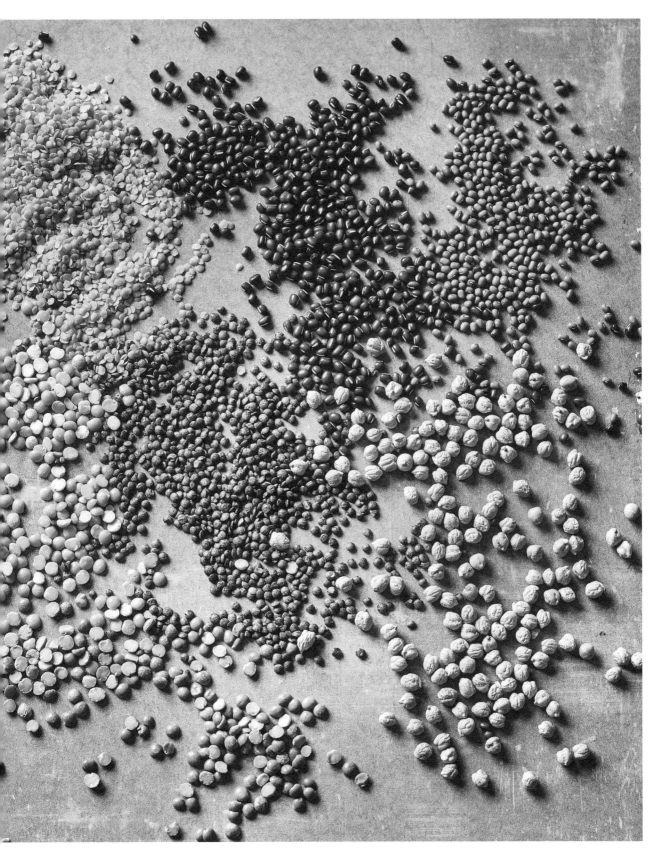

For the majority of us, however, legumes are a fantastic source of nutrition.

There are many different ways you can buy legumes. Precooked legumes in tins, packets and jars are great because they are so convenient, but the nutrient content of freshly prepared legumes is greater, and the taste and texture superior. Therefore, I try to prepare dried legumes from scratch, when I can.

The soaking times I give here are a minimum (some sources recommend soaking for longer). You should not need to drain excess water off at the end of cooking; it should all have been absorbed by the legumes. As a rule of thumb, the legumes usually double in size during the cooking process.

Mung daal, green lentils

I get a great sense of nostalgia when I cook traditional Indian dishes with these pulses. Use them for rich, hearty Indian dishes.

for 100g dried lentils

- Soak in cold water for 8–10 hours (overnight).
- Rinse thoroughly under cold running water.
- Simmer in 300ml water for 30 minutes.

French lentils, green speckled lentils, beluga lentils, puy lentils

These are by far my favourite. Their delicate, nutty flavour and slightly firm texture make them a brilliant addition to a variety of dishes.

for 100g dried lentils

- Soak in cold water for 20 minutes.
- Rinse thoroughly under cold running water.
- Simmer in 100ml water for 18 minutes.

Split yellow and green peas

I use these in mashes, coconut curries and as a side to simply cooked white fish.

for 100g dried peas

- Soak in cold water for 30 minutes–1 hour.
- Rinse thoroughly under cold running water.
- Simmer in 200ml water for 25 minutes.

Split red and yellow lentils

The easiest and quickest to cook, these lentils pair beautifully with punchy Indian flavours of ginger, chilli and cinnamon. But think outside the box too, and cook them with aromatic bay or garlic and oregano, and add them to fresh salads.

for 100g dried lentils

- Soak in cold water for 20 minutes.
- Rinse thoroughly under cold running water.
- Simmer in 200ml water for 20 minutes.

Brown daal

These take slightly longer to cook than mung daal and are regarded in Indian farming communities as a complete power food.

for 100g lentils

- Soak in cold water for 8–10 hours (overnight).
- Rinse thoroughly under cold running water.
- Simmer in 350ml water for 45 minutes.

Chickpeas and black chickpeas

Hummus made with freshly cooked chickpeas is a dip like no other. Black chickpeas are even more nutritious than the lighter variety. You can buy them online or in Indian food stores very cheaply.

for 100g dried chickpeas

- Soak in cold water for 10–12 hours (overnight).
- Rinse thoroughly under cold running water.
- Simmer in 200ml water for 30 minutes.

Kidney beans, adzuki beans, broad beans, black-eyed peas, black beans

These are fantastic in stews, soups and roasting. I like to use adzuki beans in Japanese desserts with dried fruit and berries for a delicious paste.

for 100g dried beans

- Soak in cold water for 10–12 hours (overnight).
- Rinse thoroughly under cold running water.
- Simmer in 300ml water for 45–60 minutes.

This is just a small selection of dried legumes that are available in the UK. They are a reliable source of protein and there's evidence to suggest that new, lesser-known types of beans and pulses such as lima, pinto and black beans are also really nutritious. It's an interesting avenue for future research and I would expect more unusual types of beans to be commonplace in the future as we look for more nutrient-dense sources of food to feed our growing global population.

TIP
+ The first thing I do when I get home from clinic, if I know I'm making something with dried legumes, is go to the kitchen and tip the required quantity into a big bowl of water. I do this before I even start thinking about prepping or putting the shopping away. That way, when it's time to cook I can just get on with things. Kitchen efficiency is key when you have little time.

Easy sprouting mung bean/green lentils

I find these types of lentils are the easiest to sprout. They only take a few days and it's pretty satisfying to see how they develop, but they're also widely available in supermarkets.

- Soak overnight (for at least 12 hours), until they swell up and the skins split. Rinse in a sieve under cold running water.
- Place on a tray or in a shallow bowl lined with a clean, new J-cloth or muslin.
- Store in a cool, dark place such as an empty oven or cupboard (where you won't forget about them) for 12 hours.
- Rinse in a sieve under cold running water again (you'll see some shoots emerging).
- Store in a cool, dark place again, until the shoots are 1–2cm long.
- Refresh them with water and eat them as they are, or gently sauté them with a little seasoning.

Once sprouted they will keep in an airtight container or in a bowl covered with a damp cloth in the fridge for 3–4 days. You can also freeze them for up to 8 weeks.

TIP
+ You can also sprout chickpeas and black-eyed peas, but they take slightly longer (you need to repeat the rinsing and storing process for a few more days before they germinate).

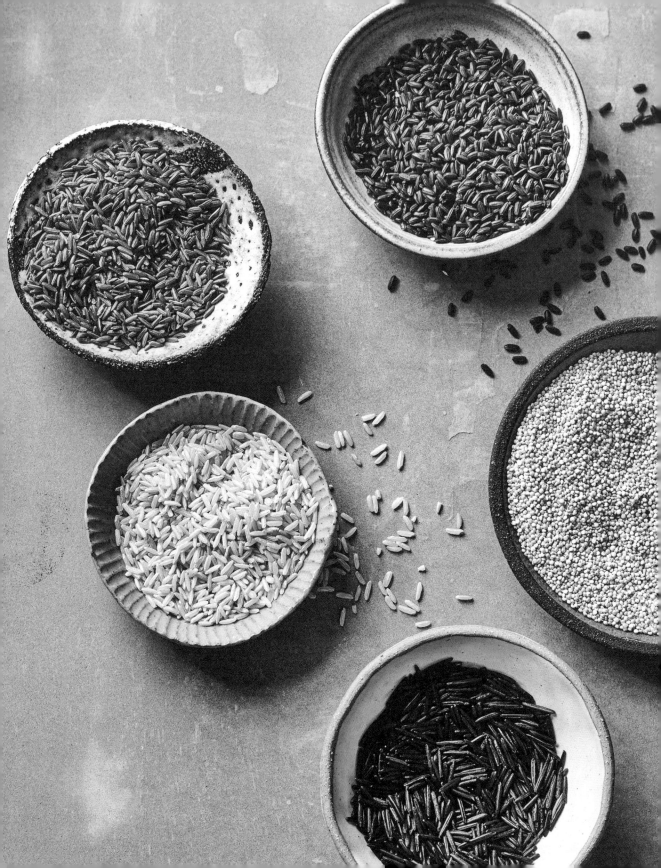

Perfect rice

I'm a big fan of incorporating rice into our diet because, in its whole form, it is a good source of fibre and phytonutrients. Eaten in the right amounts, it helps regulate blood-sugar levels and it can reduce inflammation in the body.

Again, soaking is an important step. It removes excess starch and dirt and reduces the phytate content (phytates can be an irritant to the gut). Once soaked and rinsed (see below for timings), add the rice to a hot pan and dry toast it for a minute to bring out the flavour of the grains (I sometimes do this with an oil, like coconut or extra-virgin olive oil, depending on the dish I'm preparing), then add the required amount of boiling water. Use a wide heavy-based frying pan with a lid instead of a saucepan if you can: it distributes the heat across the grains better and allows for a more even cook, resulting in fluffy, separated grains. Constantly stirring and agitating the rice when it's cooking will lead to a sticky and clumpy mixture, so when you've put the rice in the pan, leave it alone. When it's cooked remove it from the heat and leave it to stand for a few minutes with the lid on to collect its thoughts. (The only time I don't rinse rice thoroughly before cooking is when making risotto with Arborio or carnaroli rice, where the starch is needed to achieve the dish's creamy texture.)

If you know you're using a rice in a particular type of dish, season it accordingly, adding – for example – a bay leaf or a piece of fresh root ginger. Even a star anise, clove or half a citrus fruit will do wonders for flavour building.

These soaking times are a minimum (some sources recommend soaking for longer). You should not need to drain excess water off at the end of cooking, it should have all been absorbed by the grains. As rule of thumb, the grains usually increase in weight by about a half of the uncooked portion.

Red rice (French or Camargue rice)

This is by far my favourite type of rice. It cooks almost as quickly as white basmati, and the nutty flavour and texture are wonderful. The slightly increased price is worth every mouthful.

for 100g dried rice

- Soak in cold water for 20 minutes.
- Drain and rinse thoroughly under cold running water.
- Simmer, covered, in 150ml water for 14–15 minutes.

Black rice

Perhaps the most nutrient-dense rice variety. Its unmistakeable colour and nutty flavour are beautiful. I use it in sweet and savoury dishes. It's full of phytonutrients like anthocyanin that are known to be protective of the cardiovascular system.

for 100g dried rice

* Soak in cold water for 20 minutes.
* Drain and rinse thoroughly under cold running water.
* Simmer, covered, in 200ml water for 19–20 minutes.

Wild rice

This rice is wonderful and nutritious, but it takes more time to cook and it's expensive. This is my special-occasion rice and I usually use it in combination with another variety, to make it go farther.

for 100g dried rice

* Soak in cold water for 40 minutes.
* Drain and rinse thoroughly under cold running water.
* Simmer, covered, in 350ml water for 40 minutes.

Wholegrain brown rice

Despite having more health benefits than white rice, this isn't my favourite type to cook with. I sometimes find the texture too tough and starchy, but it lends itself well to desserts using coconut milk, as well as for making rice burgers and patties.

for 100g dried rice

* Soak in cold water for 20–30 minutes.
* Drain and rinse thoroughly under cold running water.
* Simmer, covered, in 250ml water for 22–5 minutes.

Quinoa

I know this isn't rice. In fact, it's not even a grain (it's a seed), but I cook it in very much the same way as rice. White, red and 'tricolour' varieties can all be cooked using this method.

for 100g dried quinoa

* Soak in cold water for 20–30 minutes.
* Drain and rinse thoroughly under cold running water.
* Simmer, covered, in 120ml water for 11–12 minutes.

Perfect potatoes

I like to put cooked sweet potato in my Tupperware for lunch as it happens to work well with many of my dishes, whether it's a lentil curry, roast fish or a pile of spicy greens in jerk sauce.

Sweet potato, purple potato, cassava, Jerusalem artichokes

Potatoes are great to cook in batches and I'll often roast or bake four or five to prepare for the week ahead. There are many types of potato but generally you can cook them all using these simple methods.

approximately 200g

Baked

- Preheat the oven to 200°C/180°C fan/gas 6.
- Scrub the skin thoroughly.
- Wrap tightly in baking paper or foil so no steam escapes.
- Bake in the oven for 45 minutes.
- Allow to cool for 5 minutes before unwrapping.
- The flesh will be soft and will come away from the skins easily (don't discard the nutritious skins — they give extra texture to mash and you can serve them as edible bowls for salads and dips).

Roast

- Preheat the oven to 200°C/180°C fan/gas 6.
- Cut into 3cm pieces (unpeeled).
- Drizzle with oil in a roasting tin, toss and season with salt and pepper.
- Roast in the oven for 35 minutes until golden.

Steam-fried

- Cut into 2cm cubes (unpeeled).
- Heat 1 tablespoon of oil in a frying pan over a medium heat.
- Add the potato cubes and sauté for 4 minutes until starting to colour.
- Splash in 30ml water and cover for 4 minutes.
- Remove lid and cook until water has evaporated.
- Serve with chopped fresh herbs such as parsley, coriander or chives.

Sides and small plates

Perfect greens

Around the UK we are so lucky to have an amazing selection of greens throughout the seasons.

We have varieties of cruciferous vegetables like broccoli and kale, not to mention the more exotic greens such as pak choy and Chinese cabbage. They are cheap, polyphenol-rich, and flavourful. Your parents were right all along: you need to eat your greens. We do not eat enough of these beautiful health-promoting plants lining supermarket shelves across the country and they are key to health. Luckily, they happen to taste delicious once you learn how to cook them properly. I lightly steam them, which preserves their vitamin content and makes them much more enjoyable to eat. These are some of my favourite seasonal greens:

Spring Asparagus, leeks, watercress, purple sprouting broccoli, spring greens, wild garlic
Summer French beans, sugar snap peas, runner beans
Autumn Chard, pak choy, broccoli, courgette, Savoy cabbage, chicory, winter cabbage, Brussels sprouts
Winter Greens, cavolo nero, pointed cabbage, kale

Brussels sprouts, cavolo nero, spring greens, winter greens, Savoy cabbage, kale (stems removed)

for 100g

- Finely chop the Brussels sprouts; shred the leaves or roll them into 'cigars' and finely chop.
- Toss into a dry frying pan over a medium heat.
- Season with salt and pepper, add 1 tbsp extra-virgin olive oil and stir for 1 minute.
- Splash in 20ml water and cover with a lid for 2 minutes.
- Uncover and make sure the water has evaporated.

Broccoli (Tenderstem), asparagus, French beans, sugar snap peas, runner beans, young kale (with stems)

for 100g

- Snap any stems in half so they fit into a pan.
- Toss into a dry pan over a medium heat.
- Season with salt and pepper, add 1 tbsp extra-virgin olive oil and stir for 1–2 minutes.
- Splash in 20ml water and cover for 2 minutes.
- Uncover and make sure the water has evaporated.

Watercress, pak choy, Swiss chard (stems removed)

for 100g

- Roughly chop the leaves.
- Toss into a dry pan over a high heat.
- Season with salt and pepper, add 1 tbsp extra-virgin olive oil and stir for 1 minute.
- Take off the heat and cover for 1 minute (the residual heat will gently wilt the leaves).

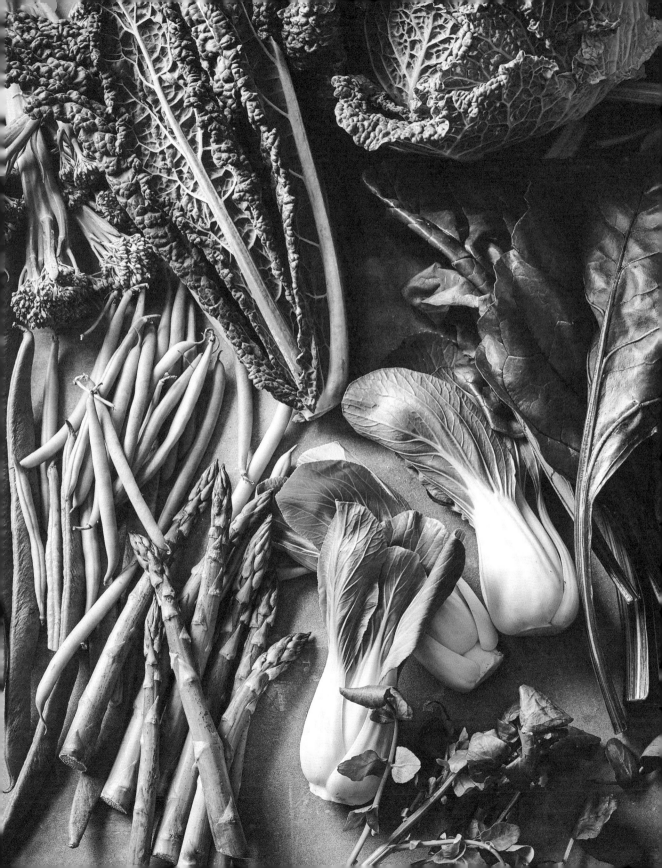

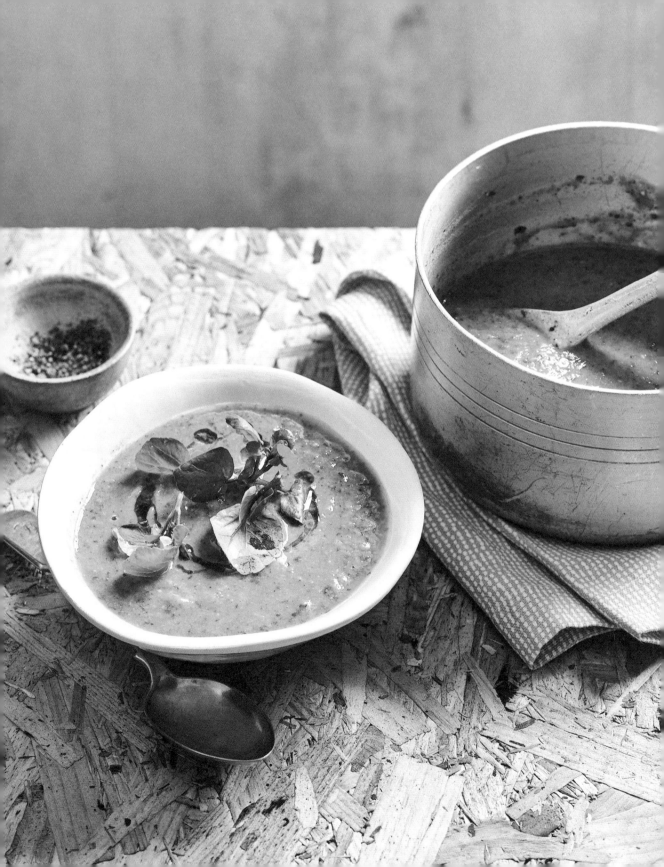

Here's a hearty spring dish that I've made even more nutritious and satisfying with the addition of split green peas. A fantastic, widely available source of protein, split peas are filling and rich in fibre. Watercress and basil may have anti-allergenic and anti-inflammatory properties, making this perfect to stock up on during the spring hayfever season. But the benefits they offer for heart health and blood-sugar stabilising alone are enough for me to recommend this dish. Enjoy the seasonal flavours and velvety texture of this glorious green soup.

Split Pea Soup with Watercress and Basil

serves 2

100g split green peas, soaked and rinsed (see page 96)

400ml boiling water

3 tbsp extra-virgin olive oil, plus extra for drizzling

3 garlic cloves, finely diced

1 spring onion, thinly sliced

200g watercress, leaves and stalks roughly chopped, plus extra to serve

25g basil leaves (about a handful), roughly chopped

sea salt and freshly ground black pepper

Put the split peas in a saucepan with half the water, place over a medium heat, bring to a simmer and cook for about 30 minutes, until mushy.

Meanwhile, heat the oil in a frying pan over a medium heat. Add the garlic and spring onion, season with salt and pepper and sauté for 2 minutes, then add the watercress and basil and sauté briefly, just for a minute or so, until wilted. Transfer to blender or food processor with the mushy split peas.

Add the remaining boiling water to the blender with the watercress and basil and blitz until smooth. Serve immediately, drizzled with extra oil, a grind of pepper and a garnish of watercress.

Sides and small plates

When I need to use up a head of broccoli in the fridge I make this dish, or variations of it. The beautiful aromas will bring everyone to the kitchen. It can be served as a simple side dish or part of a main meal with some cooked lentils and rice. Combining citrus fruit and spices with nutrient-rich greens provides extra health benefits. Roasting it whole lightly steams it, helping to retain its texture.

Whole Roast Broccoli with a Zesty Masala Dressing

serves 4

1 whole head of broccoli (about 250g), stem trimmed to give it a stable base

For the zesty masala dressing

2 oranges, 1 juiced and 1 sliced into 3cm-thick discs

2 tsp garam masala (see page 240 for my own blend)

½ tsp chilli powder

3 tbsp extra-virgin olive oil

2 tsp cumin seeds, lightly toasted

150g probiotic full-fat yoghurt

1 tsp tahini

juice of ½ lemon

sea salt and freshly ground black pepper

Preheat the oven to 200°C/180°C fan/gas 6.

Mix the orange juice, garam masala, chilli powder and oil in a bowl and season well with salt and pepper.

Place the orange discs in a single layer on a baking tray and put the broccoli upright on top of them. Pour the orange juice and spice mixture over the broccoli, cover with foil (to stop it burning) and bake in the oven for 25 minutes, then uncover and bake for a further 20 minutes, until the broccoli is lightly browned on the outside and soft inside.

Combine the toasted cumin seeds with the yoghurt, tahini, lemon juice and any roasting juices from the baking tray and dollop the yoghurt on top of the roasted broccoli to serve.

Sides and small plates

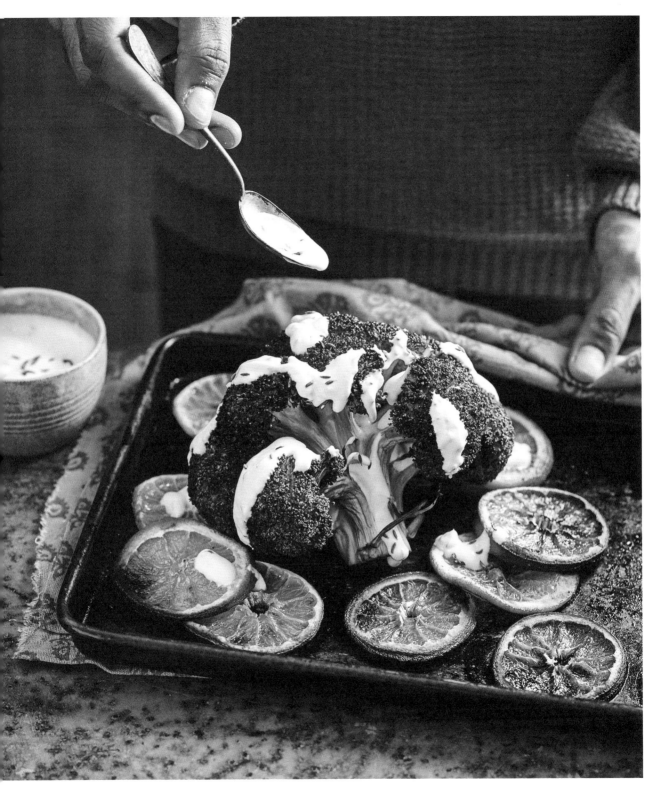

Sides and small plates

During the winter months, these are a staple in my house. They're widely available and there is a ton of research examining the health-protective effects of compounds in brassica vegetables – the list of phytochemicals in sprouts is extensive. Eat them regularly, be careful not to overcook them and pair them with lots of spices. Chestnuts, hazelnuts and good-quality extra-virgin olive oil are all fantastic ingredients that help the absorption of the fat-soluble vitamins found in these green powerhouses.

serves 2

Punchy Brussels Sprouts

2 tsp extra-virgin olive oil, plus extra to serve

2 garlic cloves, roughly chopped

1 tsp cayenne pepper

leaves from 4 thyme sprigs

200g Brussels sprouts, finely shredded

30ml water

grated zest and juice of ½ lemon

10g toasted hazelnuts, crushed

sea salt and freshly ground black pepper

Heat the olive oil in a frying pan over a medium heat, add the garlic and sauté for 2 minutes. Add the cayenne and thyme leaves and season with salt and pepper.

Toss in the shredded sprouts and cook for 1 minute, stirring, then splash in the water, cover with a lid and cook for 2 minutes. Remove the lid and make sure the water has evaporated.

Sprinkle over the lemon zest and toasted hazelnuts and drizzle with the lemon juice and some more olive oil.

TIP
+ Try this with a side of sour cream or labneh, dusted with dried chilli flakes.

Sides and small plates

I always have the ingredients to hand to make this quick side dish: peas in my freezer, garlic in the fridge door and chilli flakes in the cupboard. It goes well with lots of other ingredients such as roasted artichokes, wholewheat noodles or even a simple pesto with tomatoes and fresh mozzarella. Have this in your bank of recipes and you won't go far wrong. It offers protein from the peas, wonderful phytochemicals from the garlic and bags of flavour.

serves 2

Chilli and Garlic Peas

2 tbsp extra-virgin olive oil

2 garlic cloves, thinly sliced

200g frozen peas

1 tsp dried chilli flakes

sea salt and freshly ground black pepper

Heat the olive oil in a frying pan, add the garlic and sauté for 2 minutes.

Toss in the peas, sprinkle over the chilli flakes and season lightly with salt and pepper. Stir for 1 minute (you don't want to overcook the peas), then remove from the heat and cover with a lid for 1 minute. It is ready to serve straight away.

TIPS

+ For an aromatic twist, try adding half a star anise to the pan with the garlic. It works wonders and gives you a way to use up that jar of star anise you never use.

+ Experiment with your spice bank and see what you come up with: add cumin for an Indian twist, thyme for a British accent or rosemary and suddenly your peas are speaking Italian!

+ Fold seasonal leaves, spinach or even freshly chopped tomatoes through the finished peas to add extra flavour and colour.

Broccoli sprouts have quite a bitter flavour and the combination of them with sweet-and-salty, crispy roasted okra works so well. You'll love this sweet and sticky side dish with simple rice and broths.

Asian Okra and Broccoli Sprouts

serves 2

150g okra, cut into 2cm-thick discs

6 garlic cloves, roughly chopped

2 tbsp coconut oil

2 tbsp runny honey

1 tbsp soy sauce

50g broccoli sprouts, finely chopped (or chopped alfalfa, beansprouts or watercress)

1 tbsp unsalted peanuts or hazelnuts, dry toasted and roughly crushed

1 spring onion, finely chopped

For the dressing

1 tbsp soy sauce

3 tbsp sesame oil

2cm piece of root ginger, peeled and finely grated

½ tsp dried chilli flakes

grated zest and juice of 1 lime

Preheat the oven to 200°C/180°C fan/gas 6.

Toss the okra and garlic in a roasting tin with the coconut oil, honey and soy sauce. Roast in the oven for 12–14 minutes, until sticky and crispy.

Mix the dressing ingredients in a large bowl, add the broccoli sprouts and toss to coat. Add the sticky roasted okra and garnish with the crushed nuts and spring onion.

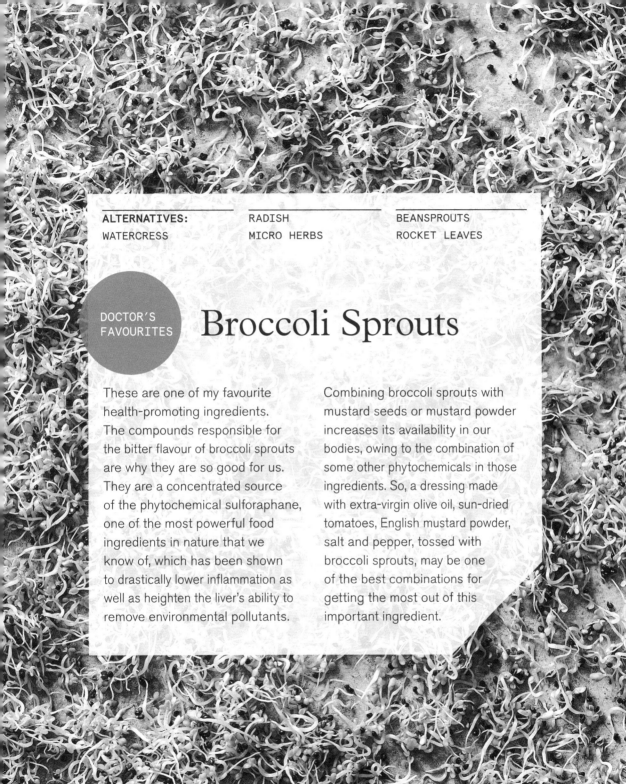

ALTERNATIVES:
WATERCRESS

RADISH
MICRO HERBS

BEANSPROUTS
ROCKET LEAVES

DOCTOR'S FAVOURITES

Broccoli Sprouts

These are one of my favourite health-promoting ingredients. The compounds responsible for the bitter flavour of broccoli sprouts are why they are so good for us. They are a concentrated source of the phytochemical sulforaphane, one of the most powerful food ingredients in nature that we know of, which has been shown to drastically lower inflammation as well as heighten the liver's ability to remove environmental pollutants.

Combining broccoli sprouts with mustard seeds or mustard powder increases its availability in our bodies, owing to the combination of some other phytochemicals in those ingredients. So, a dressing made with extra-virgin olive oil, sun-dried tomatoes, English mustard powder, salt and pepper, tossed with broccoli sprouts, may be one of the best combinations for getting the most out of this important ingredient.

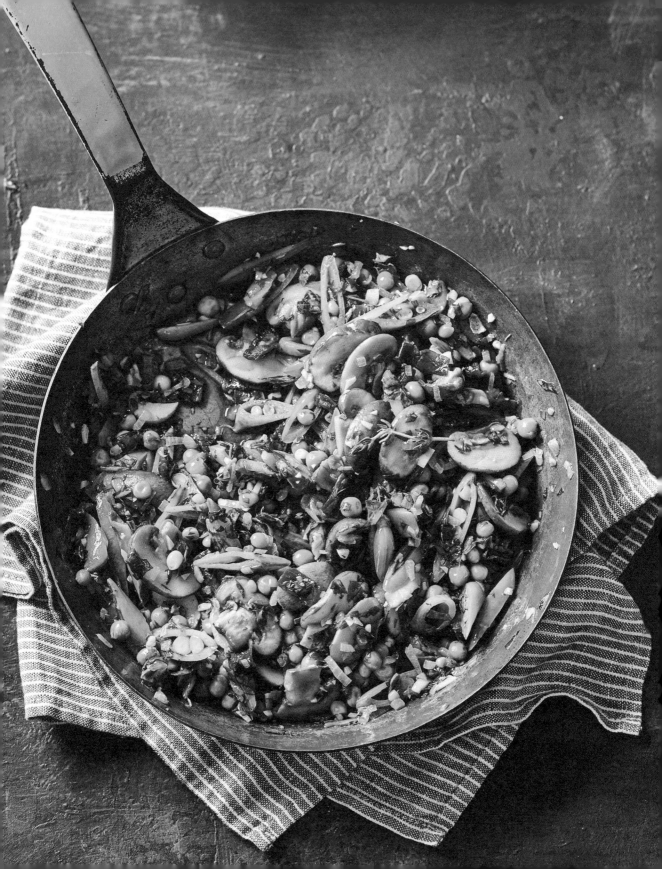

This comforting dish uses wholesome ingredients bursting with flavour. I sometimes have a big bowl of this with roasted artichokes or serve it up with leftover roast chicken. Mushrooms are a delightful source of protein and B vitamins, and sun-dried tomatoes combine with them really well.

Herby Mushrooms and Greens

serves 2

2 tbsp extra-virgin olive oil

3 shallots, finely diced

4 garlic cloves, finely diced

10g sun-dried tomatoes in oil, drained and roughly chopped

leaves from 4 thyme sprigs

50g porcini or chestnut mushrooms, thinly sliced

100g frozen peas

100g sugar snap peas, roughly chopped

50ml vegetable or chicken stock

50g spinach, finely chopped

sea salt and freshly ground black pepper

Heat the oil in a frying pan over a medium heat, add the shallots, garlic, sun-dried tomatoes and thyme and seasoning and sauté for 2 minutes. Add the mushrooms and stir gently for 2–3 minutes.

Toss in the frozen peas and sugar snap peas, pour in the stock and cook for 2 minutes. Fold through the spinach, remove from the heat and cover (the heat will gently wilt the leaves), then serve.

Sides and small plates

HEART HEALTH

The earthiness and slight sweetness of beetroot makes it a fantastic vegetable for spicing, and it works beautifully with the aromatic mixture of clove and star anise. After roasting them with freshly ground spices you won't go back to plain beetroot again! Enjoy this gorgeous antioxidant-packed vegetable with wonderful spices as a simple side dish.

serves 2

Spiced Roasted Beetroot

2 tsp coriander seeds

2 tsp cumin seeds

1 star anise

1 clove

1 tsp chilli powder

½ tsp dried chilli flakes

300g beetroot, scrubbed and cut into thick chunks

2 tbsp coconut oil, melted

sea salt and freshly ground black pepper

Preheat the oven to 200°C/180°C fan/gas 6.

Grind all the whole spices together in a pestle and mortar until coarsely ground, then stir in the chilli powder and chilli flakes.

Put the beetroot chunks in a roasting tray, toss with the melted coconut oil and ground spices and season with salt and pepper.

Cover the tray with foil, wrapping it tightly around the edges of the tray so that no steam escapes, and bake in the oven for 40 minutes.

TIP

+ Serve the roasted beetroot warm with plain yoghurt and some freshly chopped salad greens and tomatoes.

Sides and small plates

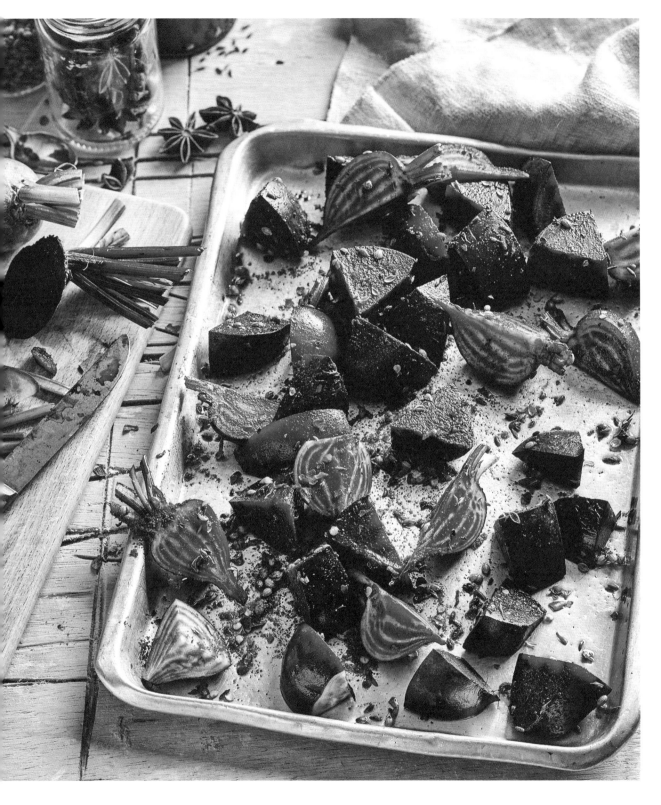

Sides and small plates

Not a fan of greens? This recipe will change your mind. Using a beautiful barbecue spice blend with added citrus and sweet notes is sure to tempt you onto this power-food dish. You can use all kinds of different greens and cabbages, such as collard greens or kale, prepped and spiced in a similar way.

Sticky Barbecue Greens

serves 2

1 tbsp runny honey

20g butter (or extra-virgin olive oil)

grated zest and juice of ¼ orange

3 tsp Best BBQ Blend (see page 243)

150g Brussels sprouts, sliced into 4mm-thick discs

150g Savoy cabbage, thinly sliced

sea salt and freshly ground black pepper

Preheat the oven to 200°C/180°C fan/gas 6.

Heat the honey in a saucepan over a medium heat. Before the honey burns, add the butter (or olive oil), orange zest and juice and seasoning and the spice blend. Simmer and reduce until it becomes sticky, then toss in the sprouts and cabbage to coat.

Tip the BBQ-coated greens onto a baking tray and bake in the oven for 12–14 minutes, until soft and glossy, then remove from the oven.

TIPS
+ You can use any other spice blend you prefer, such as harissa or even paprika with some fennel seeds.
+ Serve with plain cooked lentils or rice for a spicy delight.

Sides and small plates

This recipe uses a similar quick sriracha sauce to the one in my Sriracha Greens and Beans dish (see page 154) to create an indulgent and delicious snack that everyone will enjoy. The sweet notes of the sauce complement the sourness and chilli heat really well and the creamy aioli dip cools everything down. Egg yolks are actually quite healthy: we used to shy away from them for fear of fats, but they are a vital source of Omega-3, protein and choline, which is essential for brain health. In the context of a diet that is plentiful in plants and whole food and low in added sugar and refined carbohydrates, eggs are a great addition.

Sriracha Cauliflower Bites with Aioli

serves 2

300g cauliflower, broken into golf-ball-sized florets

3 tbsp extra-virgin olive oil

For the sriracha-style sauce

2 tbsp tomato paste

1 tbsp honey

¼ tsp cayenne pepper

1 tsp red or brown miso paste, or a pinch of salt

pinch of freshly ground black pepper

2 tsp apple cider vinegar (or white wine vinegar)

2 garlic cloves, finely chopped

3 tsp melted butter or olive oil

For the aioli

2 garlic cloves, finely grated

2 egg yolks

1 tsp wholegrain or English mustard

½ tsp sweet paprika

100ml extra-virgin olive oil

sea salt and freshly ground black pepper

Preheat the oven to 200°C/180°C fan/gas 6 and combine the ingredients for the sriracha-style sauce in a bowl.

Put the cauliflower florets in a baking tray with the oil and toss to coat. Roast in the oven for 15 minutes, until partially cooked. Remove and add the sriracha-style sauce and toss to coat the cauliflower florets. Return the cauliflower to the oven for a further 15–20 minutes until golden.

For the aioli, whisk the garlic, egg yolks, mustard and paprika in a bowl until well combined, then gradually drizzle in the oil in a steady stream, whisking continuously, until you have a thick mixture. You could also do this in a blender or food processor. Season to taste with salt and pepper.

Remove the cauliflower from the oven and leave to cool, then serve with the aioli for dipping.

TIPS

+ Try serving the aioli with crudités, such as carrots or lightly blanched asparagus.
+ Cauliflower also pairs well with my BBQ Blend (see page 243). Simply toss florets with 3 teaspoons of the blend and 4 tablespoons of olive oil, season with salt and pepper and bake for 30 minutes.

Sides and small plates

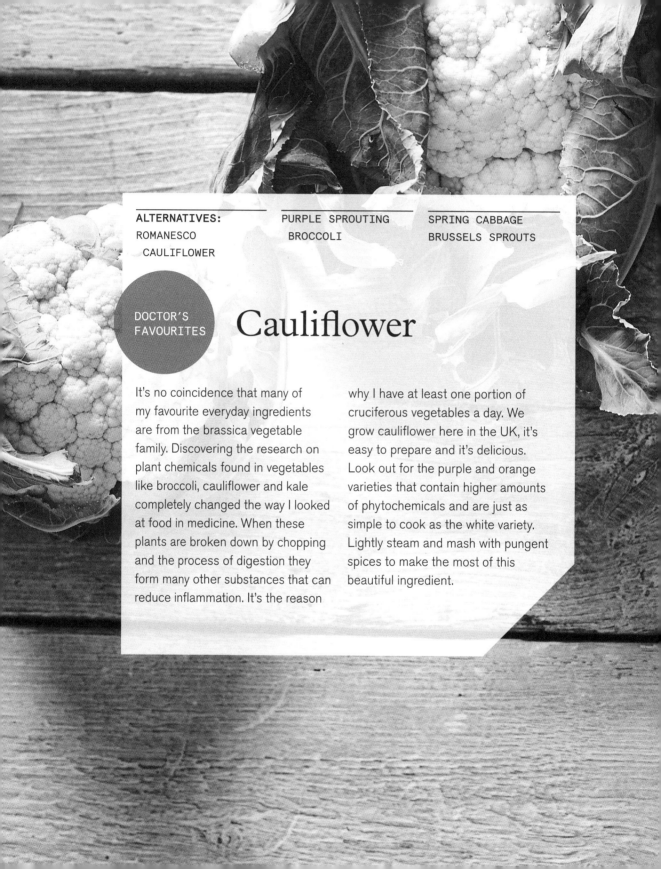

ALTERNATIVES:
ROMANESCO
CAULIFLOWER

PURPLE SPROUTING
BROCCOLI

SPRING CABBAGE
BRUSSELS SPROUTS

DOCTOR'S
FAVOURITES

Cauliflower

It's no coincidence that many of my favourite everyday ingredients are from the brassica vegetable family. Discovering the research on plant chemicals found in vegetables like broccoli, cauliflower and kale completely changed the way I looked at food in medicine. When these plants are broken down by chopping and the process of digestion they form many other substances that can reduce inflammation. It's the reason why I have at least one portion of cruciferous vegetables a day. We grow cauliflower here in the UK, it's easy to prepare and it's delicious. Look out for the purple and orange varieties that contain higher amounts of phytochemicals and are just as simple to cook as the white variety. Lightly steam and mash with pungent spices to make the most of this beautiful ingredient.

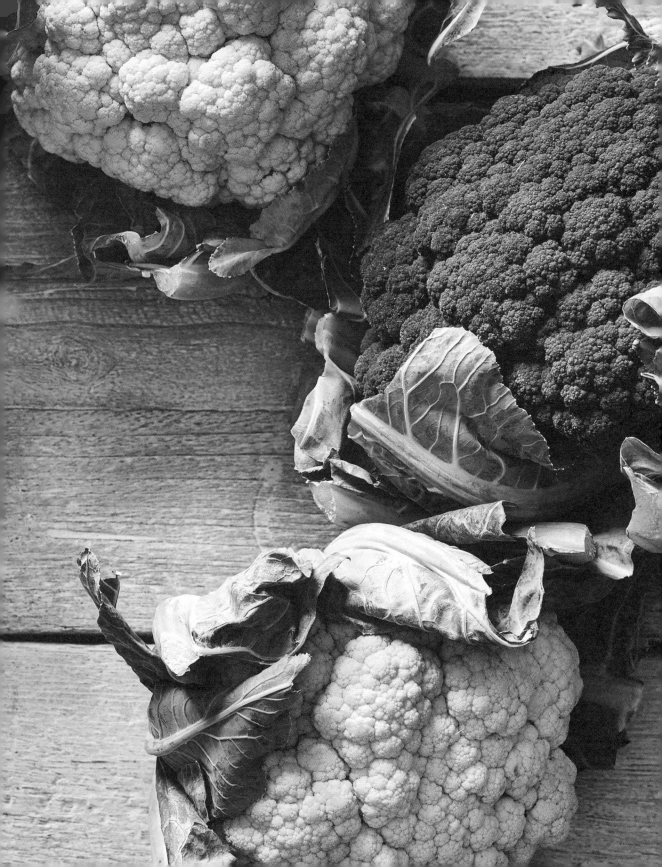

Slaws are my favourite side dish to make and the main ingredient is the humble yet phenomenal cabbage. Cheap and widely available, it is one of the most potent vegetables known to us, and it tastes fantastic with toasted fennel and lashings of extra-virgin olive oil. I like to serve this with meat or fish, or on its own with a dollop of Greek yoghurt and some toasted seeds.

Pistachio, Fennel and Red Cabbage Slaw

serves 2

200g red cabbage, finely sliced

50g rocket, finely chopped

25g parsley, leaves and stalks finely chopped

2 tsp fennel seeds, toasted

40g shelled unsalted pistachios, toasted and lightly crushed

3 tbsp extra-virgin olive oil

1 tsp dried chilli flakes

50g full-fat Greek yoghurt

juice and grated zest of ½ lemon

pinch of freshly grated or ground nutmeg (optional)

sea salt and freshly ground black pepper

Combine the cabbage, rocket, parsley, fennel seeds and pistachios in a bowl with the oil and season well with salt and pepper. Scatter over the chilli flakes.

Combine the yoghurt and lemon juice and zest, then pour it over the top, along with the nutmeg (if you wish). Stir the yoghurt through the slaw if you like a creamy coleslaw texture, and serve.

Sides and small plates

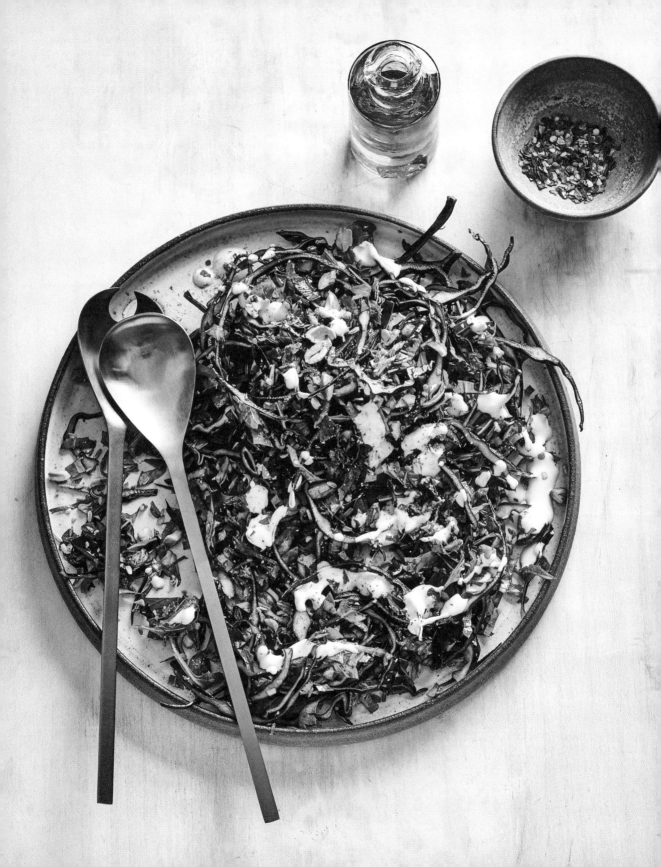

I remember the disappointment when I first ordered 'Bombay potatoes' in a restaurant in the UK. Anticipating the bright colour and flavour of what I was used to at home, I was greeted by some bland potatoes in a yellow puddle of oil. When I was young, my mother would always sneak greens into my dishes at any opportunity and I've put a twist on the classic dish by using asparagus spears. Light and crunchy, these make a welcome addition, plus they're a source of prebiotic fibre. This is a perfect side dish to complement Indian meals.

serves 2

Sweet Bombay Potatoes

3 tbsp coconut oil

1 tsp black mustard seeds

1 tsp turmeric

1 tsp garam masala (see page 240 for my own blend)

2 sweet potatoes (about 400g), cut into 2cm cubes (unpeeled)

5 asparagus spears, roughly chopped

10g coriander, stalks finely chopped, leaves retained to garnish

50ml water

sea salt and freshly ground black pepper

Melt the oil in a frying pan, add the mustard seeds, turmeric and garam masala and fry for 2 minutes until they are lightly toasted and have flavoured the oil.

Add the potatoes to the pan, season with salt and pepper and cook for 4–5 minutes until they are starting to colour. Add the asparagus and coriander stalks with the water, cover with a lid and cook for 4 minutes, until the sweet potatoes are cooked through and the asparagus is tender.

Garnish with the coriander leaves and serve immediately.

Sides and small plates

Kimchi is a probiotic, fermented food that we need to get more of into our diets. On its own it can taste quite strong, but fold it through some fresh vegetables and this Korean staple elevates any side dish. I pair kimchi with everything from chilli peas and soba noodles to poached fish, or even on its own with toasted hemp seeds. I hope this recipe will encourage you to experiment with probiotic foods, that may have gut-health benefits. The sour and fiery kimchi seasons the dish enough, so don't add more salt or soy to the mix.

Fresh Kimchi, Noodles and Shredded Cabbage

serves 2

75g kimchi

100g red cabbage, finely shredded

100g pak choy, finely shredded

50g beansprouts

80g soba noodles

25g sesame seeds

25g hemp seeds (optional)

Toss the kimchi in a bowl with the shredded cabbage, pak choy and beansprouts.

Cook the soba noodles in boiling water for 5 minutes (or according to the packet instructions), drain and fold them through the vegetables while they're still warm.

Toast the sesame seeds and hemp seeds (if using) in a dry frying pan until golden, then sprinkle them over the kimchi, noodles and shredded cabbage.

TIP
+ Sauerkraut is another probiotic ingredient that would work well in place of kimchi.

Sides and small plates

Harissa is one of my favourite spice blends. This North African combination of paprika, caraway and coriander can turn simple ingredients and dishes – cauliflower or peas, perhaps, or a simple omelette – into something quite exotic. Its unique, smoky flavour is the perfect match for celeriac, that will absorb all its tasting notes in this easy brunch dish. Celeriac is a fibre-rich root vegetable that we don't use often enough. As well as containing vitamin K and minerals, it is a source of apigenin, a plant chemical that's being examined for its ability to stop cells transforming into cancer.

Harissa, Sprout and Celeriac Fritters

serves 2
(makes 4
fritters)

100g peeled and grated celeriac

100g peeled and grated carrot

1 egg, beaten

1 tsp harissa paste

2 tsp almond flour (or any flour you have to hand – ground flax works well)

3 tbsp extra-virgin olive oil

15g broccoli sprouts, finely chopped (see Tips)

sea salt and freshly ground black pepper

Squeeze the grated celeriac and carrot over a bowl to remove excess liquid (keep the liquid). Put the squeezed-out flesh in a separate bowl along with the egg, harissa paste and flour and mix to combine.

Heat 1 tablespoon of the oil in a large frying pan over a medium heat. Take a palmful of the mixture and shape it into a fritter. Fry them in the oil in batches of 2 at a time for 2 minutes on each side, until browned and crisp. Transfer to a sheet of kitchen paper to soak up any excess oil.

Mix the sprouts in a bowl with the celeriac and carrot juices, season with salt and pepper and drizzle with the remaining oil.

Serve the fritters with the dressed sprouts.

TIPS

+ Try swapping the celeriac and carrot for different root vegetables, such as grated parsnip or sweet potato.
+ If you can't find broccoli sprouts, chopped alfalfa, beansprouts or watercress will also work well.

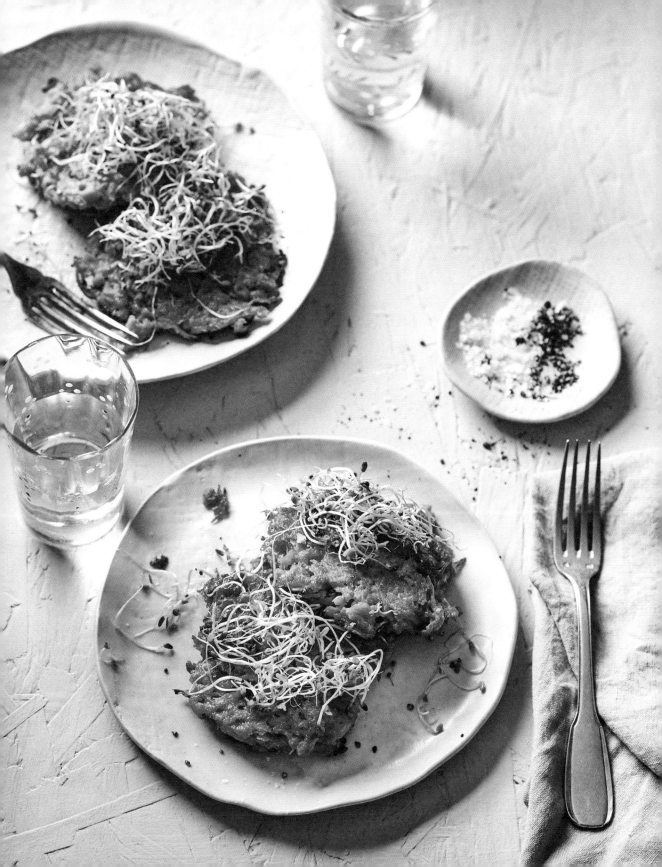

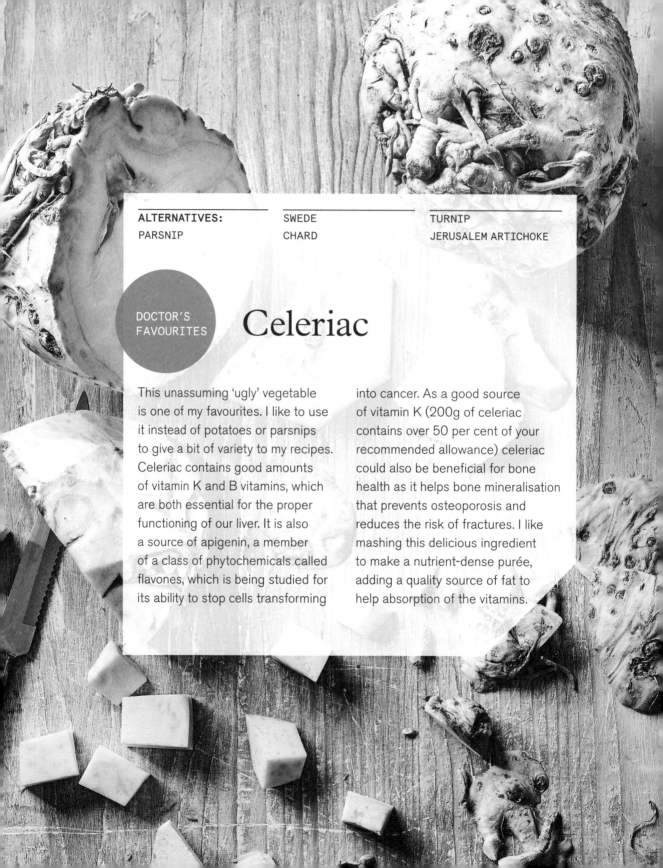

DOCTOR'S
FAVOURITES

Celeriac

This unassuming 'ugly' vegetable is one of my favourites. I like to use it instead of potatoes or parsnips to give a bit of variety to my recipes. Celeriac contains good amounts of vitamin K and B vitamins, which are both essential for the proper functioning of our liver. It is also a source of apigenin, a member of a class of phytochemicals called flavones, which is being studied for its ability to stop cells transforming into cancer. As a good source of vitamin K (200g of celeriac contains over 50 per cent of your recommended allowance) celeriac could also be beneficial for bone health as it helps bone mineralisation that prevents osteoporosis and reduces the risk of fractures. I like mashing this delicious ingredient to make a nutrient-dense purée, adding a quality source of fat to help absorption of the vitamins.

I stumbled upon the combination of spice and celeriac when designing the menu for a conference in London. I wanted to pair my homemade garam masala (see page 240) with an unusual ingredient – something earthy, creamy and delicious. Celeriac was an obvious choice. Apigenins are a type of plant chemical called flavones, which are thought to potentially reduce the incidence of cancer, and they are found in both celeriac and parsley, which just so happen to pair wonderfully in this mash. A touch of coconut and spice brings it all together, and I can guarantee it's a dish you'll keep reaching for.

Masala Celeriac Mash

serves 4

300g celeriac, peeled and cut into small 2cm cubes

50g coconut cream

2 tsp garam masala (see page 240 for my own blend)

a little coconut milk (optional)

50g flat-leaf parsley, finely chopped

salt and freshly ground black pepper

Steam the celeriac for about 12 minutes, until mushy. Transfer to a blender or food processor, add the coconut cream and garam masala, season with salt and pepper and blitz until smooth. Add a little coconut milk if necessary, to loosen it.

Transfer to a bowl, fold in the parsley, and serve.

TIP

+ Add extra coconut cream to make it even more luxurious and velvety.

I have so many memories of going to other families' houses when I was young and being greeted at the door with the familiar smell of freshly fried pakoras. The spicy, gingery aroma hit you immediately. They're a perfect match for mint chutney and, of course, masala tea. Unfortunately, these moreish snacks are far from healthy. Dunked in flour then deep-fried in poor-quality vegetable oils, they are the epitome of what's wrong with modern Indian cuisine. This recipe captures all the invigorating, nostalgic flavours of the traditional snack, but makes maximum use of good-quality, nutrient-dense ingredients. Peas are a fabulous source of protein and the chutney is a powerhouse of nutritious herbs.

serves 2

Punjabi Pakoras

For the pakoras

100g garden peas (fresh or thawed)

6cm piece of root ginger, peeled and finely grated

100g cooked puy lentils (see page 96)

100g cauliflower, coarsely grated

handful of coriander (about 20g), leaves and stalks finely chopped

3 tsp garam masala (see page 240 for my own blend)

1 tsp cumin seeds

2 tbsp coconut oil

100g spinach, roughly chopped

1 egg

sea salt and freshly ground black pepper

For the mint and coriander chutney

25g mint leaves

25g coriander (leaves and stalks)

1 green chilli, deseeded

½ apple, chopped (skin on)

150ml water

100g coconut yoghurt (optional)

Preheat the oven to 200°C/180°C fan/gas 6 and line a baking sheet with greaseproof paper.

Put all the ingredients for the pakoras in a bowl and mix by hand until well combined.

Transfer two-thirds of the pakora mix to a food processor and blitz until roughly blended (not smooth). Put the blended mixture back into the bowl with the unblended mixture, mix to combine, then shape into 6 golf-ball-sized patties.

Place the patties on the lined baking sheet and bake in the oven for 25 minutes.

While the pakoras are baking, blitz all the ingredients for the chutney (except the yoghurt) in the blender or food processor until they form a liquid mixture with some texture. Add more water if the chutney is too thick, and transfer to a bowl. Add the yoghurt to make it a milder chutney, if you wish.

Serve the warm pakoras with the chutney, for dipping.

TIPS

+ For egg-free pakoras, substitute the egg for 'flax egg': 1 tbsp ground flaxseeds combined with 3 tablespoons of cold water in a bowl and left to soak for 5 minutes.
+ Don't like cauliflower? Try grated sweet potato, celeriac or carrot.

Sides and small plates

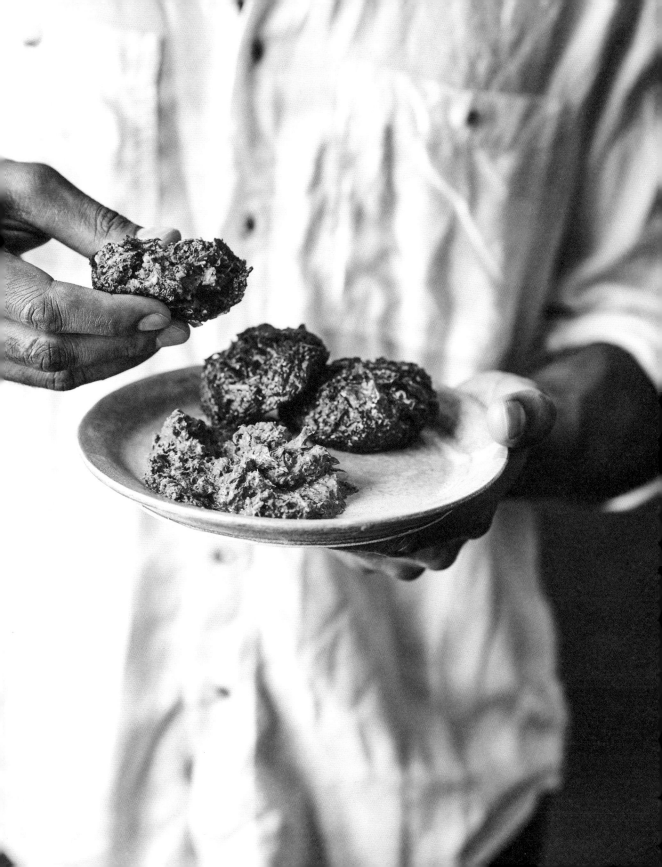

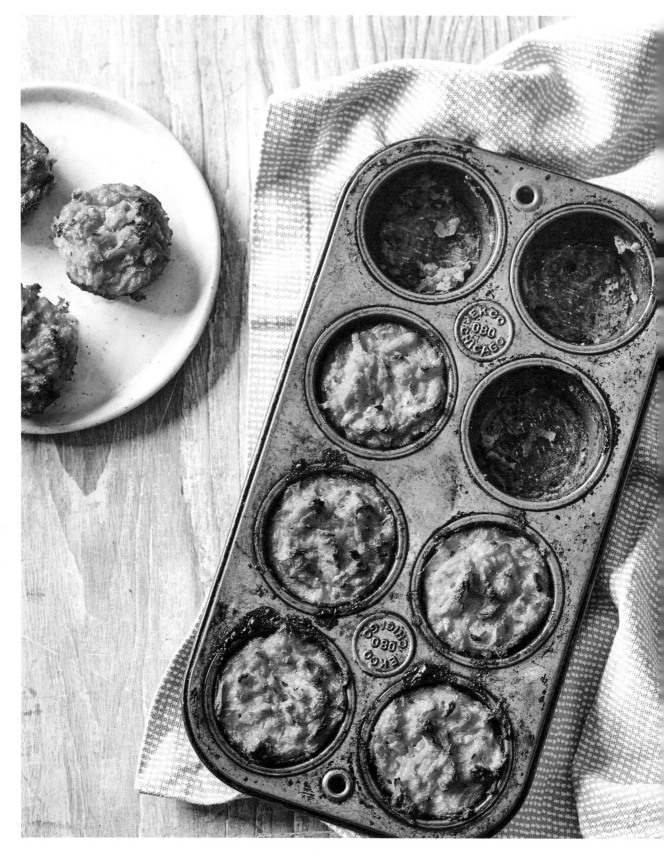

These gorgeous savoury muffins are little bites of Thailand – I enjoy them with roasted fish or even with a simple salad of spinach, peanuts and a sesame oil/fish sauce dressing. The fragrant lemongrass is a great match for celeriac, which takes on its flavour really well. I love using root vegetables in new ways, besides cooking them in simple roasts or vegetable broths.

Spicy Thai
Celeriac Muffins

makes 8
mini muffins

2 tbsp coconut oil, plus extra
　　for greasing

200g celeriac, peeled and grated

200g sweet potato, peeled
　　and grated

2 eggs

For the Thai chilli paste

5cm piece of lemongrass (tender
　　base only), thinly sliced

4 garlic cloves, roughly chopped

thumb-sized piece of root ginger,
　　peeled and roughly chopped

1 red chilli, deseeded and sliced

25g coriander stalks, chopped

3 tsp coconut cream

2 tsp soy sauce

Preheat the oven to 200°C/180°C fan/gas 6 and grease an 8-hole mini muffin tin with coconut oil.

To make the Thai chilli paste, put all the ingredients in a blender or food processor and blitz to form a rough paste.

Melt the coconut oil in a frying pan over a medium heat, add the spice paste and fry for 2 minutes, stirring, then add the grated celeriac and sweet potato and cook, stirring, for 2–3 minutes until softened.

Beat the eggs in a large bowl and add the softened celeriac and potato mixture. Stir to combine, then transfer the mixture to the muffin tin holes (a handful in each) pushing it down. Bake in the oven for 12–14 minutes, until they are browned on top.

Remove from the oven and leave to cool before removing them from the tin. They will keep in an airtight container for up to 3 days.

TIP
+ Try different vegetables in place of the celeriac and sweet potato, such as grated parsnip or even turnip.

Sides and small plates

Sometimes I want to eat something nostalgic that reminds me of my childhood, and chicken bites take me right back to school dinners. Mushrooms have a lot of benefits in the way of protein and a multitude of antioxidants, but here I'm using them in a small amount and largely as a flavour enhancer. Flaxseeds are a good source of essential fatty acids that are required for brain health, as well as fibre, and they work really well as a crumb for both chicken and fish. I enjoy these tossed through some green leaves as a snack.

Peppery Wild Mushroom Chicken Bites

serves 2

10g dried wild mushrooms

20g ground flaxseeds

2 tsp freshly ground black pepper

½ tsp cayenne pepper

a good pinch of sea salt

300g skinless chicken breasts or thighs, cut into bite-sized chunks

2 tbsp extra-virgin olive oil, plus extra for drizzling

50g snow pea shoots, roughly chopped (or finely chopped mangetout or sugar snap peas)

50g baby spinach, roughly chopped

10g pine nuts, dry toasted

Preheat the oven to 220°C/200°C fan/gas 7.

Put the dried mushrooms, ground flaxseeds, black pepper and cayenne pepper in a blender or food processor with a pinch of salt and blitz to form a fine crumb.

Coat the chicken pieces in the oil, then toss them in the spiced mushroom crumb to coat them evenly. Spread them out on a baking tray, drizzle with oil and sprinkle over some salt and bake in the oven for 14–16 minutes until cooked through, golden and crisp.

Mix the pea shoots, spinach and pine nuts in a bowl, sprinkle with a pinch of salt and drizzle with olive oil. Serve with the warm chicken bites.

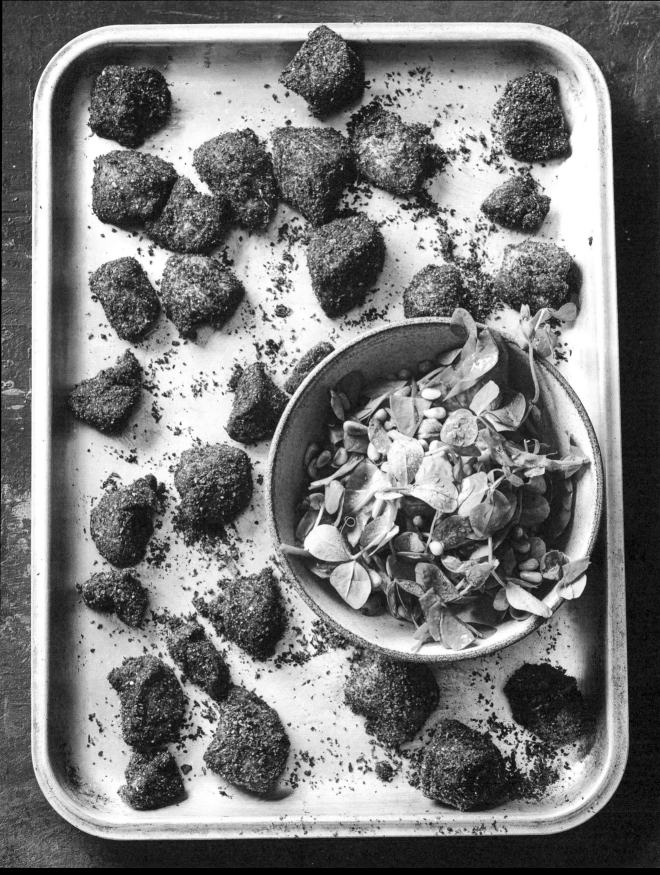

This is the first recipe I ever cooked LIVE online. I was super nervous, but loved being out of my comfort zone and channelling that nervous energy into something positive. I picked up the ingredients on my way home from work and cooked this up in less than 25 minutes. It's the most satisfying meal to end a long day in clinic. Play around with the ingredients – it's brilliant to make on a Sunday and use throughout the week for nutritious breakfasts. The broccoli stems are full of goodness, packed with fibre and minerals, and perfect for your gut health.

Facebook Frittata

serves 4

2 tbsp coconut oil

200g sweet potato, cut into 2cm cubes (unpeeled)

100g broccoli stem, trimmed and cut into 2cm cubes

½ onion, diced

3 garlic cloves, finely chopped

2 rosemary sprigs

½ tsp cumin seeds

50g kale, tough stems removed and leaves roughly chopped

½ tsp dried chilli flakes

8 eggs, beaten

sea salt and freshly ground black pepper

Preheat the oven to 200°C/180°C fan/gas 6.

Melt the coconut oil in an ovenproof frying pan over a medium heat, add the cubed sweet potato and broccoli stem and sauté for about 6 minutes, then add the onion, garlic, rosemary and cumin seeds and sauté for a further 2 minutes, until softened. Stir in the chopped kale and allow to wilt for 1 minute.

Add the chilli flakes to the beaten eggs, season with salt and pepper and pour the eggs into the pan.

Gently agitate the mixture so that the egg is evenly distributed among the vegetables and cook for 2–3 minutes, then transfer the frittata to the oven and bake for 10 minutes, until the egg has set and the top is lightly browned.

Slice and enjoy warm or cold.

TIP
+ If you can get hold of black garlic, use it in this recipe instead of regular. It's fermented garlic and it has a sweet balsamic taste which is incredible with eggs and greens. WOW.

I like to prepare these light bites when I have a bit more time on my hands and friends are popping over, and I can guarantee you're going to love them, too. I use my fiery Jerk Paste (see page 249) with peas, mushrooms and chickpeas to create fibre-rich patties, with deliciously earthy roasted beetroot adding welcome sweetness to balance the spice.

Jerk Patties 'n' Fries

makes 12 patties

For the fries

150g raw beetroot, cut into thick rounds (unpeeled)

300g sweet potato, cut into thick fries (unpeeled)

2 tbsp coconut oil, melted

For the patties

2 tsp cumin seeds

200g tinned chickpeas, drained, rinsed and dried thoroughly (or 100g dried chickpeas, cooked 'perfectly' – see page 96)

200g garden peas (fresh or thawed)

50g chestnut mushrooms, roughly chopped

3 tsp Jerk Paste (see page 249)

3 spring onions, roughly chopped

leaves from 6 thyme sprigs

3 sheets of filo (approximately 48cm x 25cm)

3 tbsp coconut oil, melted

sea salt and freshly ground black pepper

25g rocket, to serve

2 large tomatoes, thickly sliced, to serve

Toss the beetroot and sweet potato fries in a roasting tin with the 2 tablespoons of oil, sprinkle over the cumin seeds and salt and pepper and bake in the oven for 30 minutes until soft and browned.

Put all the ingredients for the patties (except the pastry and oil) in a blender or food processor and blitz to form a rough mixture.

Cut the sheets of filo in half, so you are left with approximately 12cm x 48cm sheets. Each sheet will make two patties. Using a single sheet at a time, brush the surface lightly with oil. Place a rounded teaspoon of the mixture at the short end of the strip. Fold one corner diagonally over the filling to make a triangle, flattening the filling slightly. Make two further diagonal folds and cut off (and set aside) the excess pastry. Crimp the pastry around the edges to seal and brush the top with oil. You will be left with a triangular parcel.

Put the patties in a frying pan on a low heat and fry for 2–3 minutes on each side until crisp and hot through. Alternatively, bake them at 200°C/180°C fan/gas 6 for about 12 minutes until golden.

Serve the patties with the beetroot and sweet potato fries, and some rocket and tomatoes on the side.

TIP

+ For a sweet dipping sauce, blitz some of the roasted beetroot in a blender with a garlic clove, splash of red wine vinegar, 2 tsp of tomato paste, a handful of coriander and a splash of water.

Sides and small plates

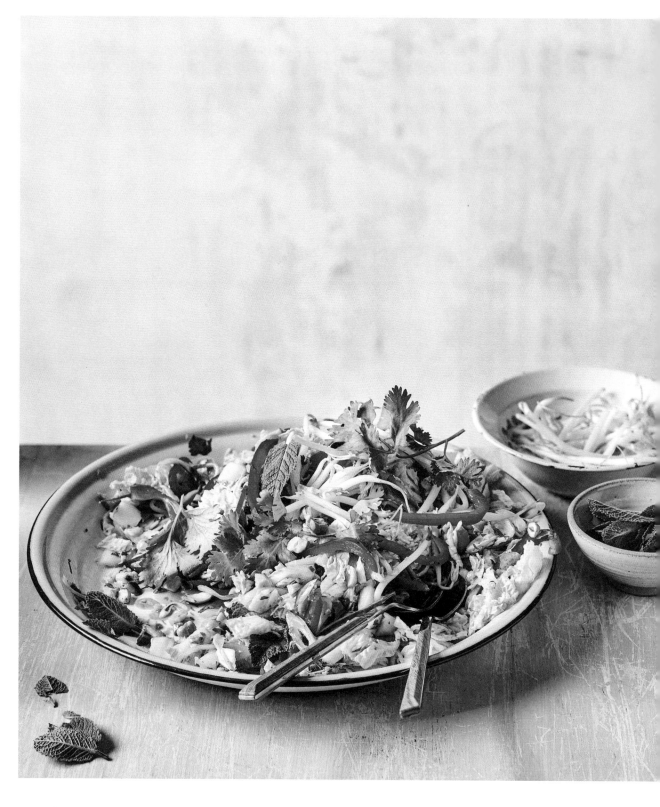

Sides and small plates

This recipe is not only absolutely smashing from a health and freshness point of view, but it brings back lots of memories for me. I had just accepted a new job in Sydney and I went to my best friend's house to tell him. He'd prepared this salad and a slow roast Massaman curry and also had some news of his own: he was relocating to Miami. It dawned on us that we were moving as far away from each other as geographically possible! The flavours in this Vietnamese dish entwine these paradoxical feelings of comfort and distance.

serves 2
with leftovers

Jay's Vietnamese Salad

For the salad

200g Chinese cabbage, finely chopped

2 spring onions, finely chopped

15cm piece of cucumber, cut into long, thin strips (unpeeled)

1 red pepper, halved, deseeded and cut into long, thin strips

15g coriander, leaves and stalks finely chopped, plus extra to serve

1 red chilli, thinly sliced

25g unsalted cashews, crushed

25g unsalted peanuts, crushed

4 mint sprigs

25g beansprouts

For the dressing

50ml sesame oil

1 tsp soy sauce

3 tsp rice wine

1 tsp dried chilli flakes

grated zest and juice of ½ lime

4cm piece of root ginger, peeled and grated

4–6 drops fish sauce (optional)

Combine the cabbage, spring onions, cucumber, red pepper, coriander and chilli in a bowl.

Toast the crushed nuts in a dry frying pan over a medium heat for a few minutes, until lightly browned, then add them to the salad.

Mix the dressing ingredients in a bowl, then drizzle it over the salad and toss to coat.

Serve the dressed salad Vietnamese-style, topped with the mint, beansprouts and fresh coriander.

TIP
+ Use 2 teaspoons of honey, maple syrup or brown sugar if you can't get hold of rice wine.

I came up with this recipe when I mistakenly overcooked some rice. I was determined not to waste the gloopy mess, so I raided my fridge for ingredients to mask the poor texture. What resulted was pure magic. Vibrant lemongrass and sharp garlic will give leftover rice (overdone or not) an amazing makeover, and prawns perfectly complement it. The Vietnamese-inspired ingredients I use in these rice balls are some of the most exciting and healthiest you can find. Also, red rice is higher in fibre and phytonutrients than white rice and not much pricier. This is a great match for Jay's Vietnamese Salad (see page 137), or simply on its own as a protein- and fibre-rich snack.

Vietnamese Prawn Rice Balls

serves 2

100g cooked camargue (red) rice (see page 99)

100g shelled raw prawns, deveined

5cm piece of lemongrass (tender base only), finely chopped, plus extra sticks (optional)

2 garlic cloves, finely chopped

10cm piece of spring onion, roughly chopped

2 tbsp coconut oil

For the dipping sauce

grated zest and juice of ½ lime

2 tbsp soy sauce

20ml sesame oil

10g sesame seeds

1 tsp honey (or palm sugar)

Put the rice, prawns, lemongrass, garlic and spring onion in a blender or food processor and blitz until just combined.

Shape the rice and prawn mixture into 4 balls (or mould them around lemongrass sticks).

Melt the coconut oil in a frying pan over a medium heat, add the prawn and rice balls (on or off the sticks) and sauté lightly for about 3 minutes on each side, until golden and cooked through. Alternatively, bake them at 200°C/180°C fan/gas 6 for about 12 minutes until golden.

To make the dipping sauce, put all the ingredients in a bowl and whisk together until combined.

TIP

+ The lemongrass skewers trick was something I picked up when I spent time in Hanoi. It's practical and infuses some flavour into the balls.

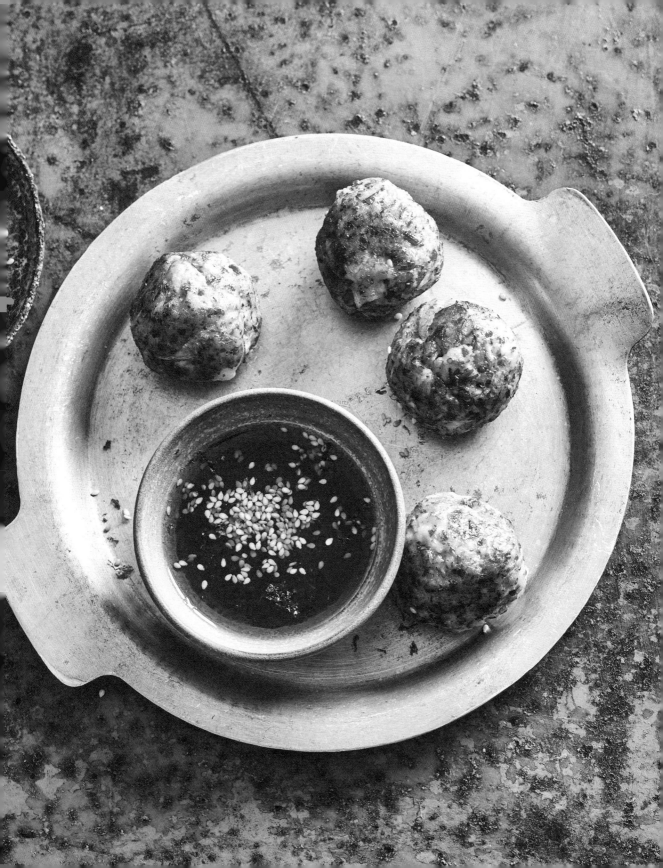

I know you want to just quickly turn the page on this one, but hear me out. Seaweed can be pungent, but weaving it into a simple side dish with other ingredients is key to acquiring a taste for it. And with the health benefits attributed to eating mineral-rich sea plants, we should at least try them. I think you'll be pleasantly surprised by this Japanese-inspired dish, rich in protein and minerals. Getting seaweed onto your plate a couple of times a week could be one of the healthiest habits you ever started.

serves 2

Seaweed Salad

3 tbsp sesame oil

3cm piece of root ginger, peeled and grated

100g Tenderstem broccoli, halved crossways

30g shiitake mushrooms, roughly chopped (enoki or chestnut mushrooms also work well)

30ml water

10g dried wakame seaweed, rehydrated in warm water for 3 minutes, then drained

1 tsp honey

1 tsp dried chilli flakes

3 tsp soy sauce

30g sesame seeds, toasted

Heat the sesame oil in a large frying pan over a medium heat, add the ginger and fry for 1 minute, then toss in the broccoli and mushrooms and cook, stirring, for 2 minutes.

Splash in the water, cover with a lid and cook for 2 minutes, then remove from the heat. Fold in the rehydrated seaweed.

Mix the honey, chilli flakes, soy sauce and sesame seeds together then toss the greens through the mixture.

TIP
+ This small plate is brilliant served with black rice.

Sides and small plates

I used to work at the paediatric emergency department in Brighton's children's hospital and I always remember the stick I got for bringing in my own trail mix! I would proudly place my jar of coconut flakes, almonds and seeds next to the packets of gummy bears and chocolate. Sugary snacks and biscuits are a common sight that keep hardworking A&E staff toiling through the day and night. I like to think I've influenced the departments I've worked in and my jars of trail mix have gently nudged co-workers to eat more nutritiously during their shifts. These are some good-quality fat and high-fibre options that I think are much better than sugary treats.

A&E Snacks

Honey and Cacao Pistachios and Cashews

makes about 100g

2 tsp cacao powder

2 tsp runny honey

1 tbsp coconut oil, melted

50g shelled, unsalted pistachios

50g unsalted cashews

Preheat the oven to 200°C/180°C fan/gas 6.

Combine all the ingredients in a bowl and ensure the nuts are thoroughly coated. Tip onto a baking tray, spread the nuts out into a single layer and bake for 14 minutes, or until the nuts are sticky and firm.

Remove from the oven and allow to cool. They will keep for up to 1 week in an airtight container.

Soy and Cayenne Seeds and Nuts

makes about 100g

2 tsp soy sauce

1 tsp cayenne pepper

1 tbsp sesame oil

50g pumpkin seeds

50g blanched almonds, skin on

Preheat the oven to 200°C/180°C fan/gas 6.

Combine all the ingredients in a bowl and ensure the seeds and nuts are thoroughly coated. Tip onto a baking tray, spread the nuts and seeds out into a single layer and bake for 14 minutes, until the almonds and seeds are toasted.

Remove from the oven and allow to cool. They will keep for up to 1 week in an airtight container.

Snacking is something I have just got used to, working in the NHS. Anyone who has worked in clinic, on hospital wards, or especially in A&E, knows how hard it is to keep to a rigid eating schedule. Although snacking isn't ideal, having a couple of nutritious and healthy bites to hand stops you going hungry or reaching for that tray of chocolate some lovely patient's family has brought in for the ward staff! These oatcakes are packed with a mixture of seeds that are fantastic sources of minerals like selenium, magnesium and zinc that have a role in supporting cell structure and may protect against heart disease. I'm no baker, but these are too easy.

Spicy Oatcakes

makes about
12 oatcakes

125g oat flour (make your own
    by pulsing 125g oats in a
    blender into a fine powder)

3 tbsp black sesame seeds

2 tsp fennel seeds, roughly ground

2 tsp cumin seeds, roughly ground

3 tbsp flaxseeds

3 tbsp pumpkin seeds

3 tbsp sunflower seeds

3 tbsp butter, softened

sea salt and freshly ground
    black pepper

Preheat the oven to 200°C/180°C fan/gas 6.

Combine all the ingredients in a bowl. Splash in a little water (about 30–50ml) and mix until the ingredients come together.

Place the mixture between two sheets of greaseproof paper and flatten it with a rolling pin to the thickness of a £1 coin.

Remove the top sheet of greaseproof paper and cut out circles or shapes roughly 5cm in diameter, place them on a non-stick or lined baking sheet and bake in the oven for 10 minutes until lightly golden.

Remove from the oven and allow to cool, then store in an airtight jar (they will keep for up to 1 week).

TIP
+ Try changing up the spices to suit your taste and using a different flour: spelt flour works well.

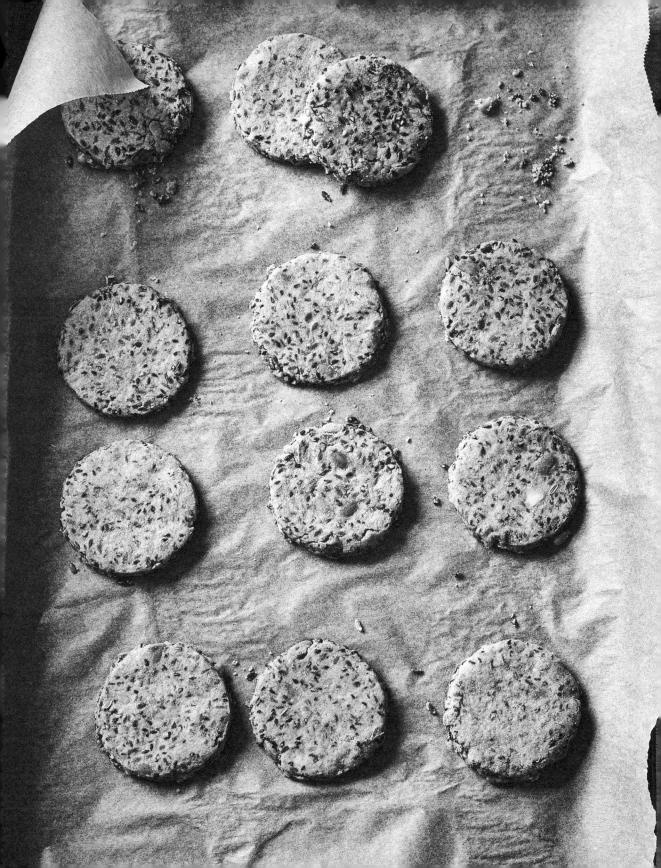

This has to be the easiest and most delicious Italian sauce I've ever tasted. My sister used to make this on 'Italian night'. (We would name days of the week according to the cuisine we'd be cooking.) Her recipe remained secret until I managed to sneak into the kitchen and see how she made it. The secret was the Worcestershire sauce! Cooked tomatoes are fantastic sources of phytochemicals and blending fresh herbs into the sauce is a great way to get used to the taste of the bitter chemicals in these nutrient-dense plants. Good-quality extra-virgin olive oil gives a wonderful Mediterranean flavour to dishes, and may also aid the absorption of the nutrients found in tomatoes.

Jasmin's Marinara Sauce

serves 2

3 tbsp extra-virgin olive oil

leaves from 2 rosemary sprigs

leaves from 2 oregano sprigs

5 garlic cloves, thinly sliced

500g passata

100g roasted red peppers (from a jar or roast your own – see Tip)

splash of Worcestershire sauce

15g flat-leaf parsley, leaves and stalks finely chopped (optional)

handful of basil leaves, torn (about 10g)

Heat the oil in a saucepan over a medium heat, add the rosemary, oregano and garlic and sauté for a few minutes until the garlic is lightly browned.

Put the passata in a blender or food processor with the roasted red peppers and blend until smooth. Add the mixture to the saucepan with the Worcestershire sauce and simmer for 5–10 minutes. Remove from the heat and stir through the parsley (if using) and torn basil leaves.

Serve warm with meatballs (see my Meatless Meatballs on page 204) or pasta dishes.

TIP

+ If you want to roast your own red peppers, halve and deseed 2 peppers, place in an oven tray skin-side up, drizzle with oil and roast in an oven preheated to 180°C/160°C fan/gas 4 for 20 minutes. Remove from the oven and leave to cool, then peel off the skin.

Sides and small plates

I love to make dips and purées with different legumes. It's so easy to experiment with different flavour combinations and whole beans are one of the healthiest ingredients you can include in your diet. Serve them with crudités, steamed vegetables or poached fish. Packed with fibre and phytonutrients, they're certainly a great, healthy alternative to bland shop-bought hummus!

Purées

serves 2

Rustic Cannellini Bean Purée

2 tbsp extra-virgin olive oil,
    plus extra for drizzling

1 shallot, finely chopped

2 garlic cloves, finely chopped

400g tin cannellini beans, drained and rinsed

4 parsley sprigs, roughly chopped

15g Roquefort cheese (optional)

30ml water

Heat 1 tablespoon of the oil in a frying pan over a medium heat. Add the shallot and garlic and sauté for about 2 minutes, until soft, then add the beans to the pan with the chopped parsley and stir for 1 minute.

Transfer to a food processor or blender, add the Roquefort (if using), water and the remaining oil, then blitz until smooth. Transfer to a dish, drizzle with oil and serve.

TIP
+ Try adding thinly sliced chestnut mushrooms when you sauté the garlic instead of cheese.

5-spice Cauliflower Purée

1 cauliflower (about 200g),
    florets roughly chopped and stem
    trimmed and chopped

2 tbsp coconut cream

100g cooked chickpeas (or 50g
    dried chickpeas, cooked
    'perfectly' – see page 96)

2 tsp Chinese 5-spice

a little coconut milk (optional)

sea salt and freshly ground
    black pepper

Steam the cauliflower for 15–20 minutes until soft, then transfer it to a blender or food processor with the coconut cream, chickpeas and 5-spice.

Season with salt and pepper and blend to a purée (adding a little coconut milk if it's too dry). Push it through a sieve to make it extra smooth, or enjoy it as it is. I prefer it rustic!

Sides and small plates

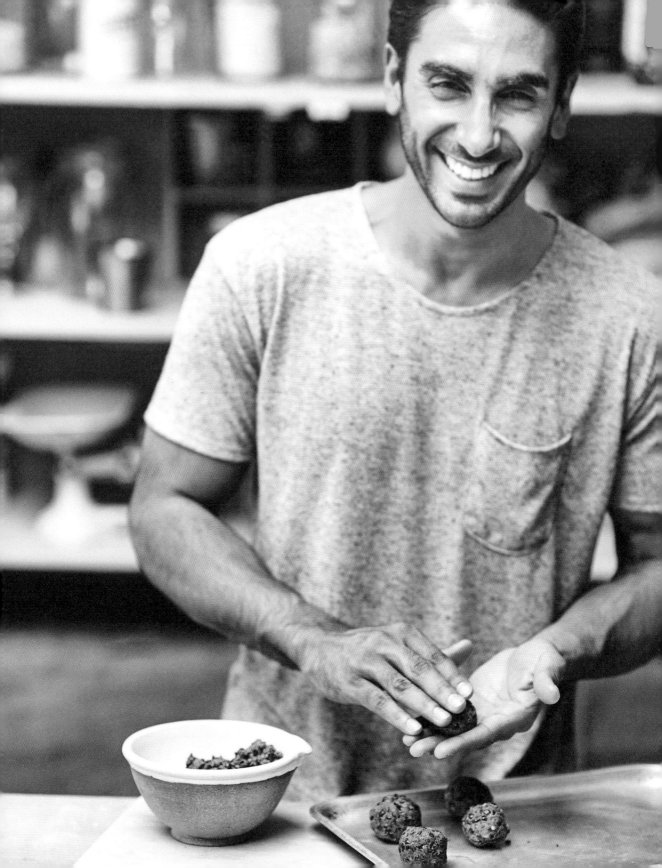

Mains

The majority of my cooking is savoury. I create lunches, dinners and things that I can easily eat the next day without too much fuss. Go off piste and experiment. Swap the ingredients for others that are in season, as they become available throughout the year. I always tend to serve dishes with a side of 'perfect greens' (see page 102) which can be made in minutes and boost the nutritional content of the meal.

A gorgeous combination of flavours, spice and medicinal properties are condensed into this warming bowl of comfort, that's simple to make and very satisfying. I start with traditional Japanese soba noodles and a simple veg broth then add layers of flavour. In their sprouted form, mung beans produce a host of active substances including vitamins and polyphenols, which is why I'm a fan of getting sprouted legumes into your diet. It's very easy to sprout beans at home and I often have them on my kitchen worktop (see page 97).

serves 2

Comforting Noodle Soup

1 tbsp coconut oil

3cm piece of root ginger, peeled and finely grated

3 garlic cloves, finely chopped

4cm piece of lemongrass, bruised

1 star anise

2 spring onions, finely chopped

350ml vegetable stock

2 tbsp soy sauce

2 tsp fish sauce (optional)

25g soba noodles

50g pak choy or spring greens, thinly sliced

25g mung bean sprouts (or snow pea, alfalfa or extra beansprouts), to serve

25g beansprouts, to serve

4 mint leaves, to serve

1 red chilli, thinly sliced, to serve

25g red cabbage, thinly sliced, to serve

Melt the coconut oil in a saucepan over a medium heat. Add the ginger, garlic, lemongrass, star anise and half the sliced spring onions and sauté for a few minutes until the garlic and onion have softened. Pour in the vegetable stock and simmer for 5 minutes.

Add the soy sauce and fish sauce (if using), then the noodles, and cook for a further 5 minutes (or according to the noodle packet instructions), until the noodles are cooked.

Remove the pan from the heat and stir through the pak choy, then leave the soup to stand for 2–3 minutes to soften the greens.

Garnish with the mung sprouts and beansprouts, remaining spring onion, mint leaves, chilli and red cabbage, and serve.

TIP

+ This recipe is really versatile: try adding different greens or vegetables – whatever you have in the fridge.

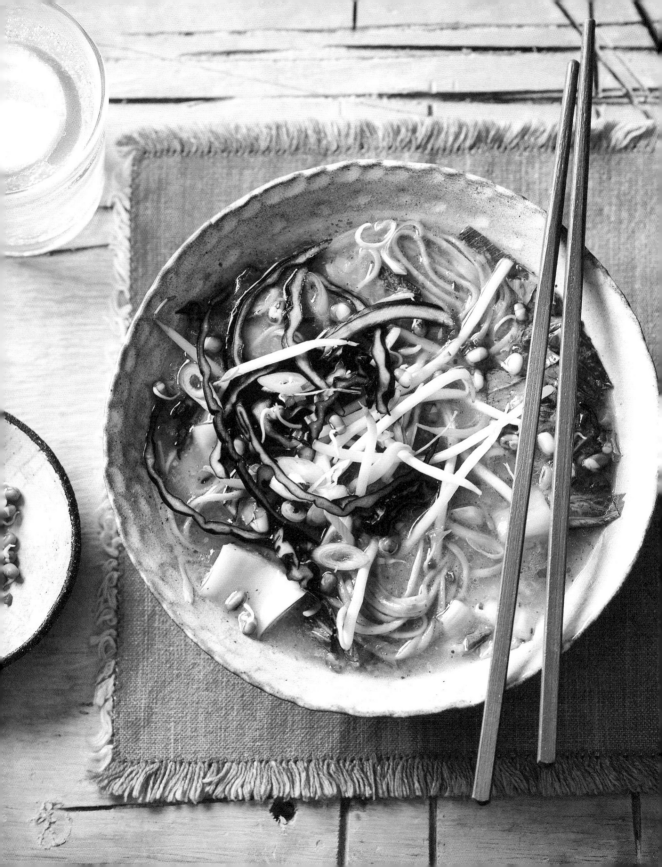

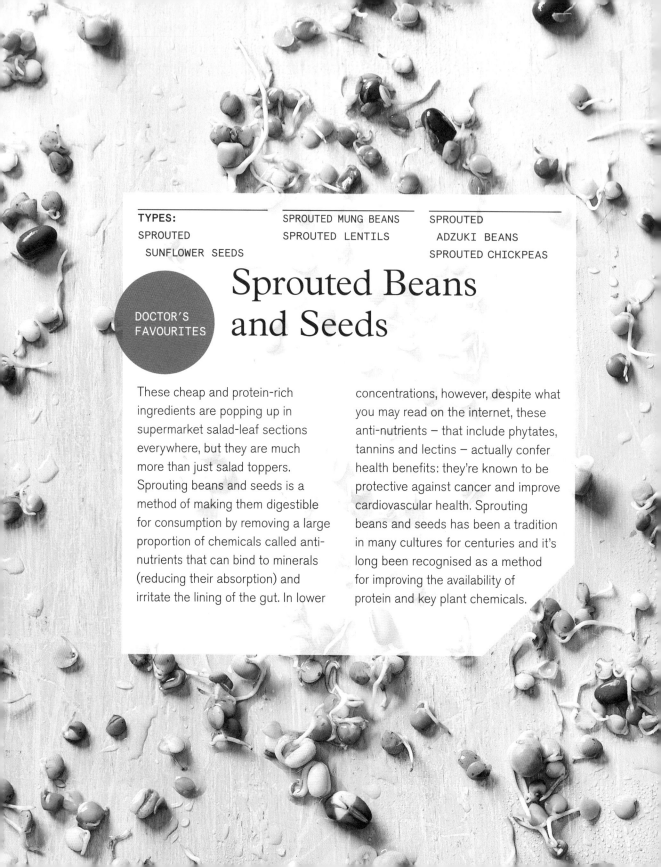

TYPES:
SPROUTED
  SUNFLOWER SEEDS

SPROUTED MUNG BEANS
SPROUTED LENTILS

SPROUTED
  ADZUKI BEANS
SPROUTED CHICKPEAS

DOCTOR'S FAVOURITES

Sprouted Beans and Seeds

These cheap and protein-rich ingredients are popping up in supermarket salad-leaf sections everywhere, but they are much more than just salad toppers. Sprouting beans and seeds is a method of making them digestible for consumption by removing a large proportion of chemicals called anti-nutrients that can bind to minerals (reducing their absorption) and irritate the lining of the gut. In lower concentrations, however, despite what you may read on the internet, these anti-nutrients – that include phytates, tannins and lectins – actually confer health benefits: they're known to be protective against cancer and improve cardiovascular health. Sprouting beans and seeds has been a tradition in many cultures for centuries and it's long been recognised as a method for improving the availability of protein and key plant chemicals.

Here's one for those veggie days, which we should all be incorporating into our weekly diet. Meat alternatives can be pretty poor, but tofu can actually taste nice. It's a bland ingredient, which is why the spicing in a tofu dish is so important. The fennel and chilli spice rub and brief grill inject it with flavour and firm it up. I tend to use extra-firm tofu here, so it'll sit nicely on this quick broth for a light meal. Get creative with fresh sprouts – they are powerhouses of nutrition.

Umami Broth with Tofu and Mung Sprouts

serves 2

3 tbsp coconut oil, melted

2 spring onions, roughly sliced

4cm piece of root ginger, peeled and finely grated

600ml chicken or vegetable stock

100g Chinese cabbage, thinly sliced

75g mung bean sprouts (or beansprouts, snow peas or thinly sliced sugar snap peas)

3 tsp brown miso paste

2 tsp fennel seeds

½ tsp dried chilli flakes, plus extra to serve

pinch of salt

200g extra-firm tofu, cut into 3cm thick rectangular slices

10cm piece of cucumber, cut into matchsticks (unpeeled), to serve

Heat 2 tablespoons of the coconut oil in a large saucepan over a medium heat, add the spring onions and ginger and sauté for 2 minutes. Add the stock and bring to the boil, then add the Chinese cabbage and half the sprouts. Remove the pan from the heat and stir the miso paste into the stock until it has dissolved. Cover and set aside for 5 minutes to allow the greens to wilt.

Put the fennel seeds and chilli flakes in a pestle and mortar with a pinch of salt and grind to a fine powder. Smother the tofu in the ground spices and coat with the rest of the melted coconut oil. Heat a dry griddle pan over a medium heat then add the tofu and grill for 3 minutes on each side until lightly charred.

Transfer the broth into serving bowls and place the grilled tofu pieces carefully on top. Garnish with the remaining mung bean sprouts, cucumber and extra dried chilli flakes.

TIP

+ Add 100g cooked black beans (see page 97, or used tinned, drained and rinsed beans) to bulk up the meal – bring them to a simmer with the stock.

In my household, as soon as anyone has a hint of a cold the pot goes on the stove and the medicinal ingredients for this broth are thrown in. Garlic, ginger, onion and chilli are well known for their anti-viral and antibacterial properties. Star anise, clove and cardamom perfume the broth, while sweet potato or squash contribute texture. Bursting with antioxidants and health-promoting properties, whenever I have a viral illness, I sip on this throughout the day. It keeps me hydrated, the strong flavours clear sinus trouble and its abundance of minerals may reduce the severity and duration of viral illnesses … It's worth a shot, as I say in clinic!

serves 4

Medicinal Broth

3 tsp butter or coconut oil

4 garlic cloves, roughly chopped

1 onion, roughly chopped

5cm piece of root ginger, peeled and grated

1 star anise

1 tsp turmeric

3 cloves

3 green cardamom pods, bruised gently in a pestle and mortar

4 bone-in chicken thighs, skin removed (optional)

300g sweet potato or butternut squash, scrubbed and cut into 4cm cubes

1 litre vegetable stock

2 tsp dried chilli flakes

50g spring greens, finely chopped

50g red cabbage, finely chopped

sea salt and freshly ground black pepper

Melt the butter or coconut oil in a large saucepan over a medium heat, add the garlic, onion, ginger, star anise, turmeric, cloves and cardamom pods and sauté for about 1 minute, then add the chicken (if using), sweet potato or squash and cook for 3–4 minutes until browned.

Pour in the stock, season with salt and pepper, add the chilli flakes and simmer for at least 20 minutes, until the chicken is cooked through and the vegetables are soft. Remove from the heat. You can cook for longer if you wish.

Add the spring greens and red cabbage to the pan, stir and cover the pan for 2 minutes to let them lightly cook, then serve.

TIPS

+ Add the fragrant chicken to rice dishes or simply remove the meat from the bone, put it in a bowl and pour over the broth to make a hearty soup.

+ Remove the chicken bones and blend the mixture with a stick blender to create a smoother soup.

I created this straight after a night shift. I wanted to make something creamy, quick and filling and despite it being 8am I didn't fancy oats! I made it with odd bits from the fridge, and my staple tin of borlotti beans turned it into a delicious meal. This soup cooks up in minutes, it's comforting, has great fibre content and pairs wonderfully with a simple side of greens and a gorgeous, fresh pesto on top. Another nod to the heart-health-promoting Mediterranean diet.

Borlotti Bean Soup

serves 2
with leftovers

2 tbsp extra-virgin olive oil

½ white onion, diced

1 celery stalk, thinly diced

2 garlic cloves, grated

1 tsp grated root ginger

leaves from 2 rosemary sprigs,
    roughly chopped

1 carrot, peeled lengthways into
    thin strips with a vegetable
    peeler, plus extra to serve

400g tin borlotti beans, drained
    and rinsed

200ml vegetable or chicken
    stock, or water

2 tbsp 'Classic Pesto', to serve
    (see page 246)

sea salt and freshly ground
    black pepper

Heat the oil in a saucepan over a medium heat, add the onion, celery, garlic, ginger, rosemary and carrot and sauté for 2 minutes, until softened.

Add the borlotti beans and stock or water, bring to a simmer and cook for 5 minutes. Transfer half the soup to a blender and blitz until roughly blended. Return to the pan and season to taste.

Alternatively, roughly blitz the mixture in the pan with a stick blender or masher until you have a rustic soup texture.

Serve topped with the pesto and a few carrot strips.

TIPS
+ You can use white, cannellini or even butter beans.
+ Homemade pesto tastes far superior, but there's nothing wrong with store-bought if you're short of time.

The Korean flavours of sriracha sauce and chilli-fermented cabbage were a revelation to me. I remember the first time I ate authentic Korean fried chicken. The sticky, sweet crispy wings were paired with the most amazing chilli and pickle flavours. I want you to experience the same taste sensation without the trans fats and sugar! Proper kimchi is another gut-healthy food that tastes wonderful folded through rich greens. Broad beans are perfect in summer and they're a great source of protein and fibre. The 'fried' egg on top pays homage to the classic Korean presentation. My sriracha-style sauce needs acidity, sweetness and heat. You should have most of the sauce ingredients in your cupboard.

serves 2

Sriracha Greens and Beans

100g red rice, soaked in cold water for 20 minutes, drained and rinsed

2 tsp coconut oil

100g podded broad beans

150g kale, tough stems removed and leaves roughly chopped

1 romano red pepper, deseeded and roughly chopped

4 pak choy leaves, torn

2 eggs

50g kimchi

1 tsp sesame seeds, toasted

For the quick sriracha-style sauce

3 tbsp tomato paste

1 tbsp honey

½ tsp cayenne pepper

1 tbsp red miso paste or soy sauce

pinch of freshly ground black pepper

1 tbsp apple cider vinegar (or white wine vinegar)

1 tsp garlic paste (or 2 grated garlic cloves)

splash of water

Simmer the rice in 150ml of water for 14–15 minutes.

Meanwhile, combine the ingredients for the sriracha-style sauce in a bowl and set aside. Preheat the grill to medium.

Melt 1 teaspoon of the coconut oil in a frying pan over a medium heat, toss in the beans and cook for 2–3 minutes. Add the chopped kale, red pepper and pak choy and cook for a further 2 minutes, then mix in the sriracha-style sauce, cover and cook for 1 minute before removing from the heat.

Melt the remaining coconut oil in a separate frying pan over a medium heat, crack in the eggs and when they start to turn white on the top, place under the grill for 2 minutes, until the whites are cooked but the yolks are still runny.

Pile the sriracha greens onto the rice, add the kimchi, top with the fried eggs and sprinkle with the toasted sesame seeds.

TIP

+ You can save some of the sriracha sauce to fold through the rice before serving.

Mains

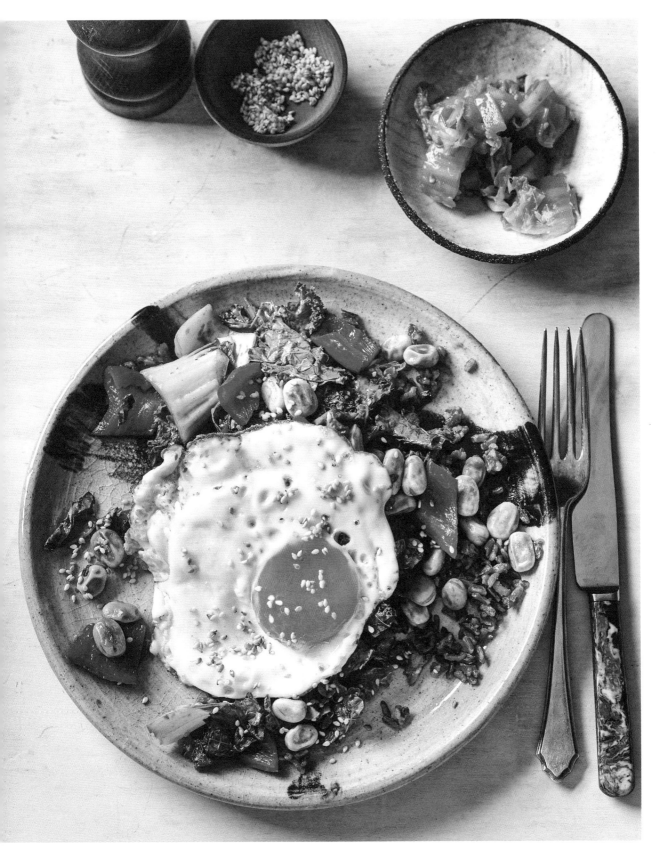

One of the lessons I was taught growing up in my Indian household was the importance of flavouring hot oil or ghee with spices before adding the bulk of the ingredients. This process ensures we appreciate the full impact of the spices and creates incredible aromas that permeate through the dish. Welcome to healthy, rapid Indian cooking! This traditional gobi (which means cauliflower) is loaded with inflammation-fighting brassica vegetables, along with medicinal spices and a really nutrient-dense salad.

Colourful Gobi

serves 2

2 tbsp ghee, butter or coconut oil

1 tsp black mustard seeds

1 tsp garam masala (see page 240 for my own blend), plus extra to serve

1 star anise

thumb-sized piece of root ginger, peeled and grated

head of cauliflower (about 250g), florets roughly chopped

1 trimmed broccoli stem (about 100g), cut into 3cm cubes (keep the florets for another dish)

1 sweet potato (about 150g), cut into 2cm cubes (unpeeled)

25g coriander, leaves picked (for garnish) and stems finely chopped

15g dried fenugreek leaves (optional)

50ml boiling water

sea salt and freshly ground black pepper

100g kefir, coconut yoghurt or full-fat probiotic yoghurt, to serve

cooked red rice (see page 99) or traditional wholemeal Indian bread, to serve

For the traditional Indian salad

½ red onion, thinly sliced

1 cucumber, sliced lengthways into thin strips

1 green chilli, deseeded and finely chopped

½ lemon

Melt the ghee, butter or coconut oil in a large frying pan over a low heat, add the mustard seeds, garam masala, seasoning and star anise and toast them for 1–2 minutes until fragrant. Add the ginger and sauté for a further minute, then add the chopped cauliflower, cubed broccoli stem and sweet potato and cook for 5 minutes, until softened. Add the coriander stems, dried fenugreek leaves (if using) and boiling water. Cover and cook for 6–8 minutes, until the vegetables are tender but not mushy.

To make the traditional Indian salad, combine the red onion, cucumber and green chilli in a bowl and squeeze over the juice from the lemon.

Garnish the gobi with the coriander leaves and serve with the salad, bread or rice and the yoghurt of your choice, sprinkled with garam masala.

Tofu is a versatile, protein-rich ingredient and a source of isoflavones that are known to reduce the incidence of cancer and improve bone health. I try to include soya in my meals a couple of times a week, and particularly enjoy the taste and firm texture of smoked tofu: it's much more appetising than raw tofu. I promise you'll love the complement of greens in this dish.

Smoked Tofu Greens

serves 2

50g brown rice noodles

2 tbsp coconut oil

3 garlic cloves, finely chopped

3cm piece of root ginger, peeled and finely chopped

50g pak choy, thinly sliced

50g Chinese cabbage, finely shredded

100g smoked tofu, cut into 2cm slices

1 tsp honey

2 tbsp soy sauce

grated zest and juice of 1 lime

1 red chilli, finely chopped (deseeded if you wish)

1 garlic clove, finely grated

10g dry roasted peanuts, roughly crushed

3 mint leaves, roughly torn

Put the brown rice noodles in a heatproof bowl, immerse in boiling water, cover and leave to soak for 6–8 minutes (or according to the packet instructions), then drain.

While the noodles are soaking, melt the coconut oil in a large frying pan over a medium heat, add the garlic and ginger and sauté for 1–2 minutes until lightly coloured. Toss in the pak choy and Chinese cabbage and fry for 2 minutes, stirring, until lightly wilted. Add the smoked tofu pieces and cook for 2 minutes, stirring, to warm it through.

Whisk the honey, soy sauce, lime zest and juice, chilli and grated garlic together in a bowl, then stir it into the tofu and greens and cook for 1 minute.

Garnish the smoked tofu greens with the peanuts and fresh mint, and serve with the drained noodles.

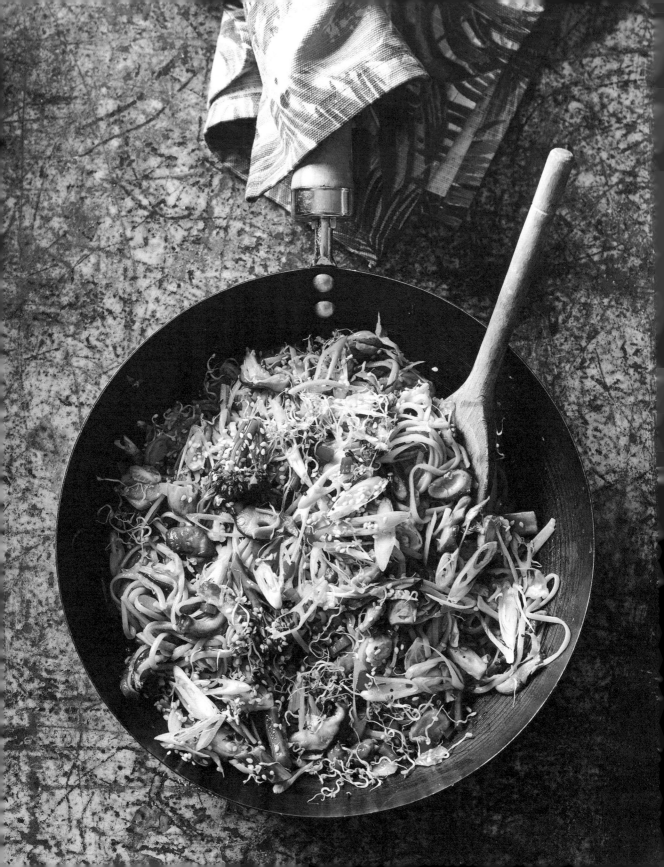

A simple paste of garlic and ginger with a splash of soy sauce makes this fiery Asian fusion dish burst with flavour. Shiitake mushrooms give it substance, but you can easily replace them with chestnut mushrooms. Broccoli and broccoli sprouts are a source of the phytochemical sulforaphane, one of the most powerful natural food ingredients that we know of. The broccoli sprouts have a bitter mustard bite to them, which makes them a perfect garnish.

Japanese Mushrooms with Purple Broccoli and Rice Noodles

serves 2

100g brown rice noodles

1 tbsp coconut oil

100g baby Brussels sprouts, thinly sliced

100g shiitake mushrooms, thinly sliced

100g purple Tenderstem broccoli, roughly chopped (or regular Tenderstem if purple is out of season)

1 spring onion, thinly sliced, to serve

25g broccoli sprouts, washed and dried (or beansprouts, finely chopped pea shoots or rocket), to serve

10g sesame seeds, toasted, to serve

1 red chilli, deseeded and thinly sliced, to serve

For the paste

1 shallot, roughly chopped

2cm piece of root ginger, peeled and grated

2 garlic cloves, roughly chopped

2 tbsp soy sauce

Put the brown rice noodles in a heatproof bowl, immerse in boiling water, cover and leave to soak for 6–8 minutes (or according to the packet instructions), then drain.

While the noodles are soaking, put the paste ingredients in a blender or food processor and blitz until roughly blended, adding a little water if needed, to loosen.

Melt the coconut oil in a frying pan over a medium heat, add the paste and fry for 1 minute, then add the sliced Brussels sprouts and mushrooms to the pan. Cook for 2 minutes, then add the broccoli with a splash of water (about 25ml). Cover and cook for 2 minutes.

Stir the cooked and drained noodles through the vegetables, then remove from the heat and serve, garnished with the spring onion, broccoli sprouts, sesame seeds and chilli.

TIP

+ If you can get hold of a Japanese paste called koji, mix 1 teaspoon of it with the ginger and garlic paste for an even more authentic umami flavour.

Black beans are used so innovatively in Japanese cuisine, in both sweet and savoury dishes. I wanted to create something that celebrates the bean's versatility, so came up with this easy stew. The umami sauce made with miso paste and coconut oil gives it a unique flavour, and may have positive effects on our gut health. The sauce pairs very well with the beans and takes seasonal veggies on a culinary journey to the Far East. Despite miso's high sodium content, it doesn't appear to have a detrimental effect on blood pressure – scientists have hypothesised that this may be due to the relative high antioxidant component. (If you are concerned about salt intake, speak to your doctor about consuming miso; it may not be something to have on a regular basis.)

Miso Black Bean Stew

serves 4

4 tbsp coconut oil

1 leek (about 200g), washed, trimmed and roughly chopped

200g asparagus spears, trimmed and roughly chopped

200g kale, tough stems removed and leaves roughly chopped

400g cooked black beans (200g dried black beans, cooked 'perfectly' – see page 97 – or 400g tin black beans, drained and rinsed)

2 tsp brown miso paste

fresh spinach salad or cooked wild rice (see page 100), to serve

Melt 2 tablespoons of the oil in a large frying pan over a medium heat, add the leek, asparagus and kale and sauté for about 3 minutes. Stir in the black beans to heat through.

Mix the miso paste with the remaining oil and 100ml hot (not boiling) water, and dress the vegetables and beans in the umami sauce.

Enjoy with a fresh spinach salad or side dish of wild rice.

I spent part of my medical elective at a human genetics research lab in the University of California in San Diego. We were so close to Mexico that my friends and I decided to head south in search of adventure. I was glad I convinced them to let me go to Oaxaca, as I wanted to try a dish called mole where they use raw chocolate to create an unbelievable savoury sauce. Its sweet, bitter notes with fiery chilli make a novel yet comforting combination. I use flavanol-rich cacao with vegetables to create my version. Don't be put off by using chocolate in a savoury dish – it works perfectly with the sweet tomatoes and corn.

serves 4

Mexican Mole

1 sweetcorn cob (or 100g tinned sweetcorn)

4 tbsp extra-virgin olive oil

1 red onion, finely diced

4 garlic cloves, finely chopped

1 tsp cumin seeds

1 bay leaf

1 tsp cayenne pepper

1 dried ancho chilli, deseeded (or 1 tsp dried chilli flakes or chipotle dried chilli flakes)

200g sweet potato, cut into 3cm cubes (unpeeled)

400g tin kidney beans, drained and rinsed (or 200g dried kidney beans, cooked 'perfectly' – see page 97)

200g passata

1 tbsp cacao powder (or good-quality 100% cocoa powder)

50g spring greens, finely chopped

50g red cabbage, finely shredded

sea salt and freshly ground black pepper

50g French beans, cooked 'perfectly' (see page 102), to serve

Grate the sweetcorn cob into a bowl using a box grater. It should be liquid and creamy.

Heat the olive oil in a saucepan over a medium heat, add the onion, garlic, cumin seeds, bay leaf, cayenne and ancho chilli or chilli flakes. Season with salt and pepper and sauté for 2 minutes, until the onion is soft but not browned. Add the cubed sweet potato and cook for 2–3 minutes, until softened, then add the grated (or tinned) sweetcorn and kidney beans and stir. Tip in the passata with the cacao powder, stir again, cover and simmer for 10 minutes.

Stir in the spring greens and red cabbage for the last 2 minutes to lightly cook them.

Serve the mole with the green beans.

TIP
+ This meal also goes well with a side of cooked white quinoa.

Fish sauce is a pungent, unmistakeably Southeast Asian ingredient that I love using. It gives Thai curries a restaurant quality, and used sparingly, it's a brilliant seasoning for cruciferous vegetables. These simple noodles, dressed with oil, garlic and ginger, are all you need to hit your senses, and the synergistic effects of different antioxidants in these ingredients may be more powerful than previously thought. The nuts and gorgeous greens give this light and easy-to-prepare dish bags of protein and fibre.

Soy Roasted Vegetables with Ginger Noodles

serves 2

3 tbsp coconut oil, melted

½ tsp turmeric

2 tbsp soy sauce

½ tsp chilli powder

150g broccoli, separated into 3cm florets, and stem trimmed and diced

150g cauliflower, separated into 3cm florets (keep the leaves)

1 red onion, roughly cut into chunks

80g buckwheat soba or brown noodles

25g sugar snap peas, thinly sliced

25g spinach, finely chopped

10g unsalted peanuts, crushed

lime wedges, to serve

1 red chilli, sliced, to serve

For the dressing

5cm piece of root ginger, peeled and finely grated

1 garlic clove, finely grated

30ml sesame oil

2 drops of fish sauce (optional)

Preheat the oven to 200°C/180°C fan/gas 6.

Mix the melted coconut oil, turmeric, soy sauce and chilli powder together in a bowl. Put the broccoli, cauliflower and onion in a separate large bowl, add the coconut oil mixture and smother the vegetables in it. Tip the vegetables into a roasting tray and bake for 25 minutes, until golden.

Meanwhile, mix the dressing ingredients together in a large bowl and cook the noodles in a pan of boiling salted water for 6 minutes (or according to the packet instructions). Drain the noodles, then transfer them to a large serving bowl. Add the sugar snap peas and spinach and half the dressing and toss to combine.

When the vegetables are cooked, remove them from the oven and tip them straight into the bowl with the remainder of the dressing, while they're still hot.

Serve the noodles with the roasted and dressed vegetables on top, scattered with the peanuts, with lime wedges and sliced red chilli on the side.

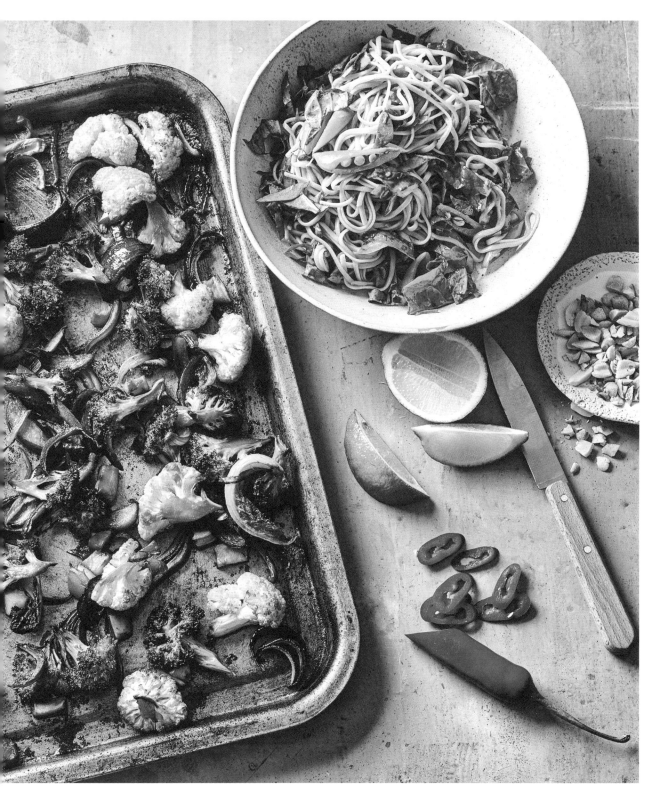

Mains

My friends couldn't believe the food I ate at home after school. My mother would experiment with different cuisines and use my sister and I as taste testers. We loved it. Our ultimate favourite was chilli garlic prawns in lashings of extra-virgin olive oil soaked up with freshly baked baguette. The kitchen would smell glorious with the marriage of garlic and shellfish. Mum made it look effortless … because it is! Try this beautiful recipe to which I've added a few extra ingredients. Phytonutrients are most concentrated in the skins of vegetables so try to leave the skin on when possible.

serves 2

Mum's Chilli Garlic Prawns

1 courgette, peeled lengthways into thin strips with a vegetable peeler

1 yellow pepper, halved, deseeded and cut into matchsticks

1 raddichio (about 75g), finely chopped

4 tbsp extra-virgin olive oil

4 garlic cloves, very finely chopped

250g shelled raw jumbo prawns, deveined

1 tsp dried chilli flakes

sea salt and freshly ground black pepper

5–6 basil leaves, torn, to serve

cooked wholegrain pasta, sourdough bread or 'steam-fried perfect' potatoes (see page 101), to serve

Combine the prepared vegetables in a bowl.

Heat the olive oil in a frying pan over a low heat, add the garlic and fry until lightly browned, then place the prawns in the pan and season with salt and pepper – the prawns should sizzle, but the pan should not be so hot that the oil splutters.

Fry for 2 minutes, then turn the prawns over and add the chilli flakes to the pan and continue frying until the prawns are cooked through. Transfer them to the bowl of vegetables and pour the flavoured oil from the pan over the top.

Garnish with the torn basil leaves and serve with wholegrain pasta, toasted sourdough bread or potatoes.

TIPS

+ For an extra herby flavour, add a sprig of thyme to the oil when you add the chilli flakes and take it off the heat. Allow it to infuse its flavour for a minute, then drizzle it onto the vegetables.
+ Raddichio is a vibrant source of essential prebiotic fibre, but endive or simple lettuce also work well.

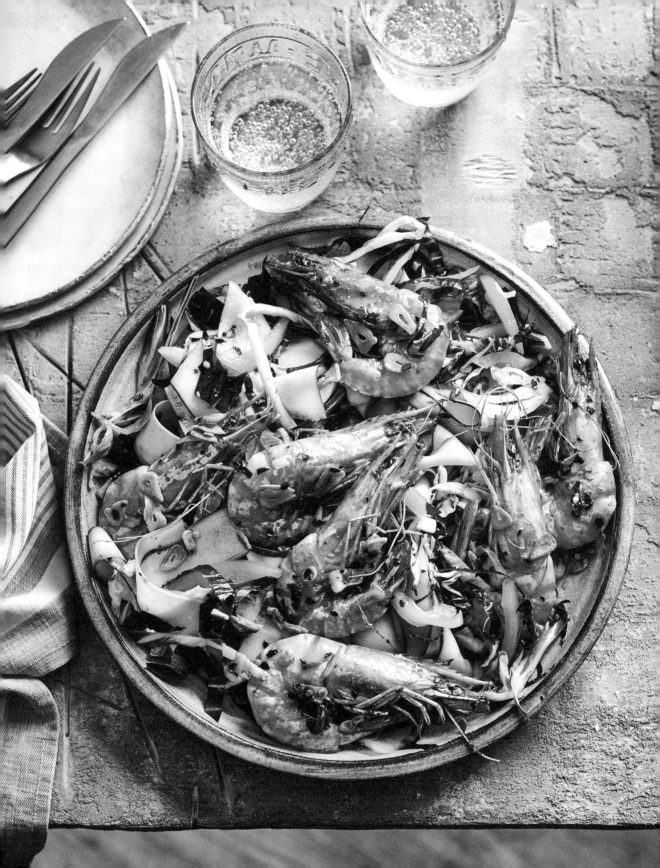

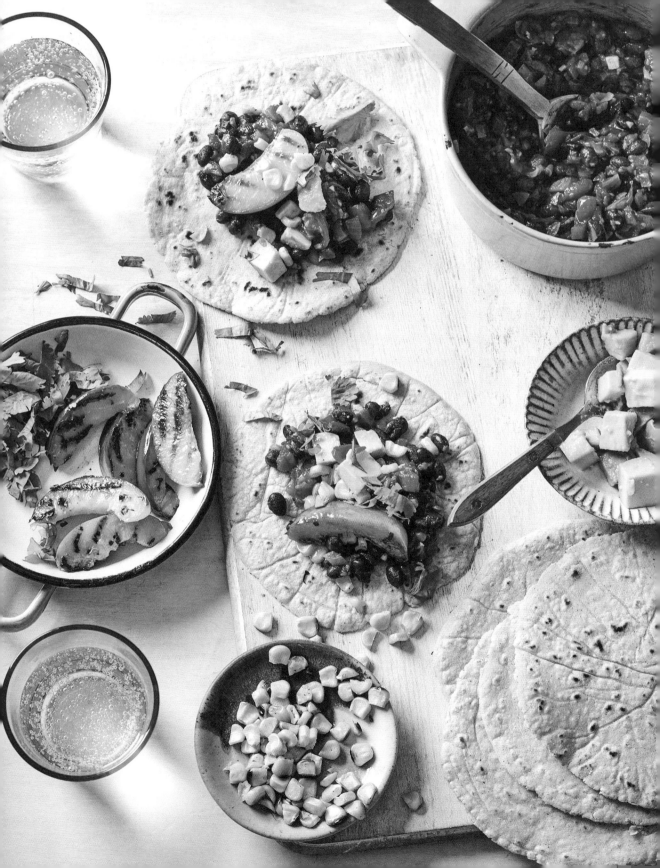

I love this recipe, it makes including a great range of colours in one meal really achievable – vibrant colours are key to good health and this recipe has an abundance of them. Mexican food is one of the healthiest and easiest cuisines to replicate at home, once you remove the unnecessary fried ingredients and processed cheese. This dish is light and the ancho chillies pack a fruity punch that's perfect with the grilled sweet nectarines. You can buy corn tortillas but making them from scratch is very simple (see page 168).

Black Bean Tacos with Grilled Nectarine

serves 2

2 tbsp extra-virgin olive oil, plus extra for brushing

4 garlic cloves, finely chopped

1 red onion, diced

1 dried ancho chilli, soaked in 100ml hot water for 10 minutes, then deseeded

2 tbsp tomato paste

400g tin black beans, drained and rinsed (or 200g dried black beans, cooked 'perfectly' – see page 97)

2 ripe nectarines, stoned and cut into thick wedges

1 sweetcorn cob (or 100g tinned kernels, rinsed)

4 corn tortillas (shop-bought or see recipe on page 168)

1 ripe avocado, stoned, peeled and diced

handful of coriander, chopped

½ lime

sea salt and freshly ground black pepper

Heat the oil in a saucepan over a medium heat, add the garlic and red onion and sauté for a few minutes until softened.

Put the ancho chilli and its soaking water in a blender with the tomato paste and blitz until smooth.

Add the black beans to the onion and garlic with the blended chilli and tomato paste and simmer for 5 minutes.

Meanwhile, brush the nectarine wedges and sweetcorn cob with oil, place on a hot griddle pan, turning frequently, until lightly charred all over. The nectarines only need 2–3 minutes. Grill the sweetcorn cobs for a further 2–3 minutes until tender.

Slice the kernels off the grilled corn cob. Build your tacos with the grilled corn (or tinned corn) and nectarine, avocado and black beans, garnish with the coriander and a squeeze of lime.

TIPS

+ This recipe works well with any stone fruit, such as apricot and peach.
+ Buy a smoky chipotle paste if you can't find dried ancho chillies.

I learnt to make these when I visited Mexico on my medical elective. Their simplicity was revolutionary – it's essentially how we make traditional *makki di roti* (a type of Punjabi bread). Masa Harina is a type of gluten-free flour made from ground corn or cornmeal. You can find it online and it's definitely worth seeking out if you want to make authentic corn tortillas.

Homemade Tortillas

makes 4

100g Masa Harina flour

pinch of salt

150ml cold water

Mix the flour and salt in a bowl, add the water and mix to form a smooth dough that holds its shape. Continue to add water a little at a time, if necessary, until you get the desired texture, or add more flour if the dough is too sticky.

Divide the dough into 4 small balls, cover with a sheet of baking parchment and use the base of a frying pan to press them down on the worktop into 10–12cm rounds a few millimetres thick.

Heat a dry frying pan or griddle pan over a high heat until hot, then add a tortilla and cook it for about 2 minutes on each side until lightly coloured. Remove from the heat and cook the remaining tortillas. Allow to cool and stack them up to serve.

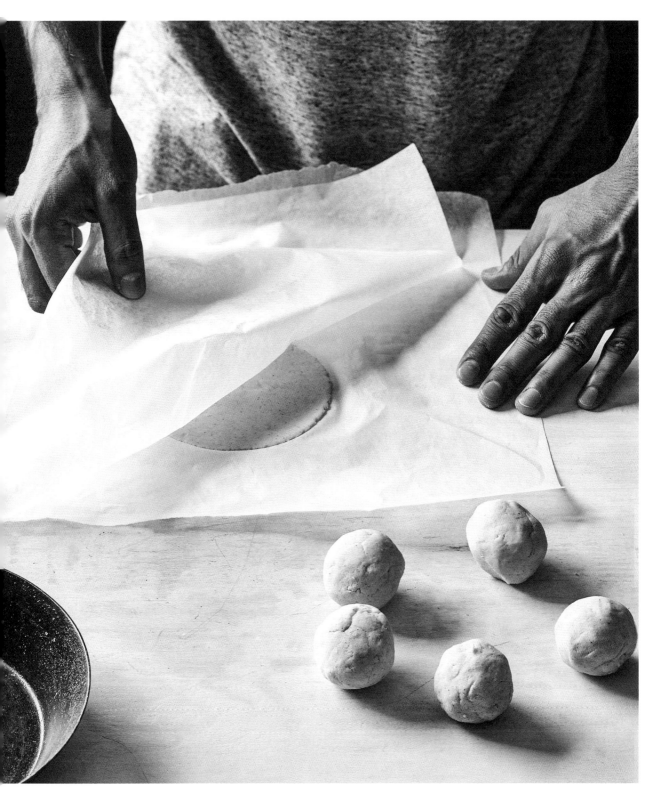

Mains

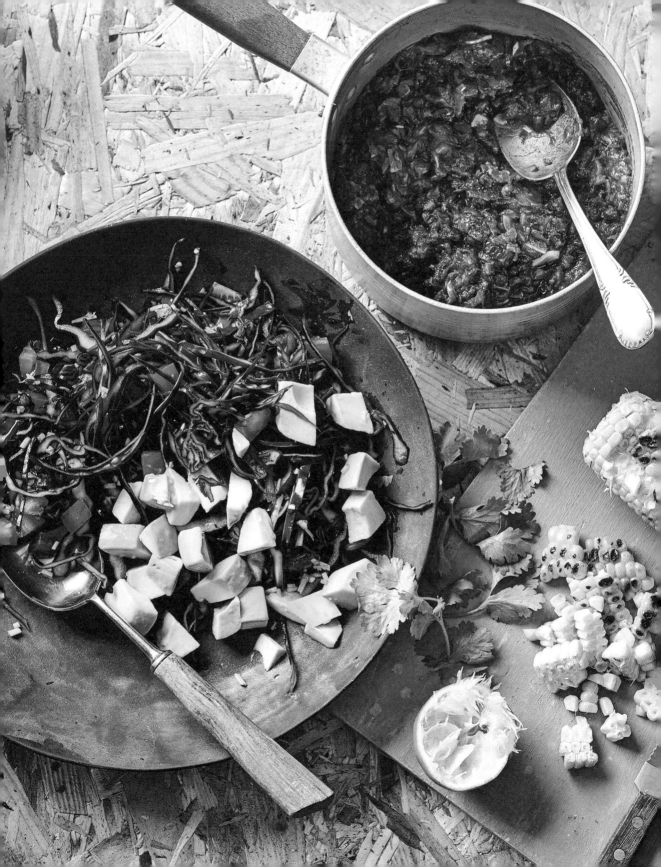

Mexican cuisine is as vibrant and colourful as the country! Remove the typical breads, wraps and cheeses that are low in nutrients and load up on the spice, fresh vegetables and healthy fats. We grow delicious sweetcorn in the UK (look out for it in late summer). If there was one dish that represents how I believe we should eat more often, it's this Mexican bowl, bursting with colour, lots of fibre and good-quality fats.

Mexican Black Bean Chilli Bowl

serves 4

4 tbsp extra-virgin olive oil, plus extra for drizzling

3 garlic cloves, thinly sliced

1 red onion, finely diced

1 tsp smoked sweet paprika

1 tsp dried chilli flakes

1 tsp cumin seeds

400g tin black beans, drained and rinsed (or 200g dried black beans, cooked 'perfectly' – see page 97)

2 large tomatoes, finely diced

1 tsp runny honey

3 sun-dried tomatoes in oil, drained

2 sweetcorn cobs (or 200g tinned sweetcorn, drained)

150g red cabbage, finely shredded

1 ripe avocado, stoned, peeled and diced

10g coriander, leaves and stalks separated and finely chopped

grated zest and juice of 1 lime

sea salt and freshly ground black pepper

Heat 2 tablespoons of the oil in a saucepan over a medium heat, add the garlic, onion, paprika, chilli flakes and cumin seeds, season with salt and pepper and sauté for 2 minutes, then add the black beans and cook, stirring, for a further 2 minutes.

Put half the tomatoes in a blender or food processor with the honey, the remaining oil and the sun-dried tomatoes and blitz until smooth. Add the mixture to the pan of beans and simmer for 8–10 minutes.

If you're using whole corn cobs, coat them in a drizzle of oil, a little salt and pepper and grill under the oven grill or on a griddle pan, turning them frequently, until tender and lightly charred all over.

Mix the shredded red cabbage in a bowl with the remaining diced tomato, avocado and coriander stalks.

Slice the corn kernels off the cob straight into the bowl of cabbage (or add the drained tinned sweetcorn) with the lime juice and zest and a drizzle of oil.

Serve the bean stew on top of the vegetables in the bowl, and garnish with the coriander leaves.

TIP
+ This pairs well with a portion of cooked wholegrain rice.

Wild rice and lentils are the perfect combination. This is a take on kitchari, a traditional Indian dish, but I use different flavours and wholegrain rice (instead of refined white basmati rice) for its added fibre, protein and taste. A simple switch from white to wholegrain rice has been shown to improve sugar levels in diabetics and I honestly think it tastes much better. You become satiated quicker and the nutty puy lentils pair well with firmer rice. The mellow flavours of bay and thyme anglicise this dish, but feel free to add a hint of chilli if you wish.

Wild Rice and Puy Lentils with Broccoli

serves 2

3 tbsp extra-virgin olive oil

2 bay leaves

1 red onion, finely chopped

4 thyme sprigs

3 garlic cloves, finely chopped

200g wild red (or brown) rice, soaked for at least 20 minutes, then drained

200g puy lentils, soaked for 20 minutes, then drained

600ml boiling water

200g Tenderstem broccoli

2 tbsp tahini

juice and zest of 1 lime

sea salt and freshly ground black pepper

10g flat-leaf parsley, leaves roughly chopped and stalks finely chopped, to serve

Heat 2 tablespoons of olive oil in a saucepan over a medium heat, add the bay leaves, onion, thyme and garlic and sauté for a few minutes until lightly browned.

Add the rice and lentils and toast them in the oil for 1–2 minutes, to infuse the flavours, then pour in the boiling water, cover and simmer for at least 20 minutes, until the lentils and rice are cooked but still al dente.

While the rice and lentils are cooking, cook the broccoli. Toss the stems into a dry pan over a medium heat, season with salt and pepper, add the remaining olive oil and stir for 1–2 minutes. Splash in 40–50ml water and cover with a lid for 2 minutes.

Uncover and make sure the water has evaporated, then transfer to a bowl. Combine the tahini, lime juice and zest and 10ml boiling water in a bowl to make a dressing and drizzle it over the broccoli.

Serve the rice and lentils with the broccoli and garnish with chopped parsley.

TIP

+ Add dried chilli flakes to the rice and lentils, to give them a kick, if you like, or add ½ teaspoon of ground cinnamon or a clove to the pan at the start, to give it a more aromatic flavour (as well as additional antioxidant value).

Mains

Sometimes the best meals are made by throwing some good-quality spices at some good-quality ingredients that take on flavour really well. This is the sort of meal I make after a long day in clinic. No fuss or mess, but tons of nutrition. Chipotle is a gorgeous smoked jalapeno chilli with a medium heat. I use chilli quite often in cooking, largely to add flavour, but it's interesting that the active chemical capsaicin in chilli is being investigated for its ability to reduce inflammation and promote cardiac health in patients with angina.

Chipotle Beans, Spicy Quinoa and Grilled Sweetcorn

serves 2
with leftovers

2 tbsp extra-virgin olive oil

2 garlic cloves, finely diced

½ red onion, finely diced

1 tsp chipotle chilli powder, plus extra to serve

1 tsp sweet paprika

100g peas (fresh or thawed)

200g podded broad beans

100g white quinoa, soaked in cold water for 20–30 minutes, then drained and rinsed

150ml water

1 sweetcorn cob, halved widthways

grated zest and juice of 1 lime

sea salt and freshly ground black pepper

Heat the oil in a frying pan over a medium heat, add the garlic, onion and spices, season with salt and pepper and sauté for 2 minutes until softened. Add the peas, broad beans and rinsed quinoa and toast them in the oil for 2 minutes, then pour in the water and cook for 12 minutes, or until the water has been absorbed.

Meanwhile, grill the sweetcorn cob halves for 6 minutes on each side under a medium grill or on a griddle pan until cooked and lightly charred all over.

Dress the quinoa and grilled sweetcorn with the lime juice, some salt and a sprinkle of extra chipotle chilli powder.

I first tried these chicken balls while cycling through Vietnam and the flavour was mesmerising. The fragrant lemongrass is unmistakeable, and the dish is brought together by a gorgeous salad which makes full use of incredibly healthy Thai ingredients including ginger, garlic and lime. A touch of sugar helps balance out the saltiness of the soy and fish sauce. You shouldn't be scared of sugar. We need to hugely reduce our intake but that shouldn't be at the expense of enjoying food where it is a helpful addition.

Vietnamese Chicken and Lemongrass Balls with Mangetout and Carrot Salad

serves 2

1 tbsp coconut oil

For the chicken and lemongrass balls

5cm piece of lemongrass (tender base only), finely chopped

2 tsp coconut cream

2 garlic cloves, roughly chopped

5cm piece of root ginger, peeled and finely grated

2 tbsp soy sauce

1 spring onion, finely chopped

small bunch of coriander, leaves and stalks finely chopped

300g skinless chicken breast, cut into chunks

50g chestnut mushrooms, chopped

For the dressing

30ml sesame oil

1 tsp fish sauce

3 tsp soy sauce

1 tsp sugar

grated zest and juice of 1 lime

1 garlic clove, grated

4cm piece of root ginger, peeled and finely grated

1 tsp dried chilli flakes

For the salad

50g mangetout, thinly sliced

2 carrots, peeled lengthways into thin strips with a vegetable peeler

10g unsalted, toasted peanuts, roughly crushed

Preheat the oven to 200°C/180°C fan/gas 6 and grease a baking tray with the coconut oil.

Put the lemongrass, coconut cream, garlic, grated ginger, soy sauce, spring onion and coriander in a blender or food processor and blitz to form a rough paste. Add the chicken and mushrooms and blitz again until roughly chopped.

Tip the mixture into a bowl, form it into 4 golf-ball-sized rounds, place the balls on the greased tray and bake in the oven for 12 minutes, until browned and cooked through.

Meanwhile, whisk the dressing ingredients together in a bowl.

Toss the mangetout and carrot strips in a bowl with some of the dressing, sprinkle in the peanuts, and put the rest of the dressing in a shallow bowl for dipping the chicken and lemongrass balls into.

Serve with perfectly cooked rice.

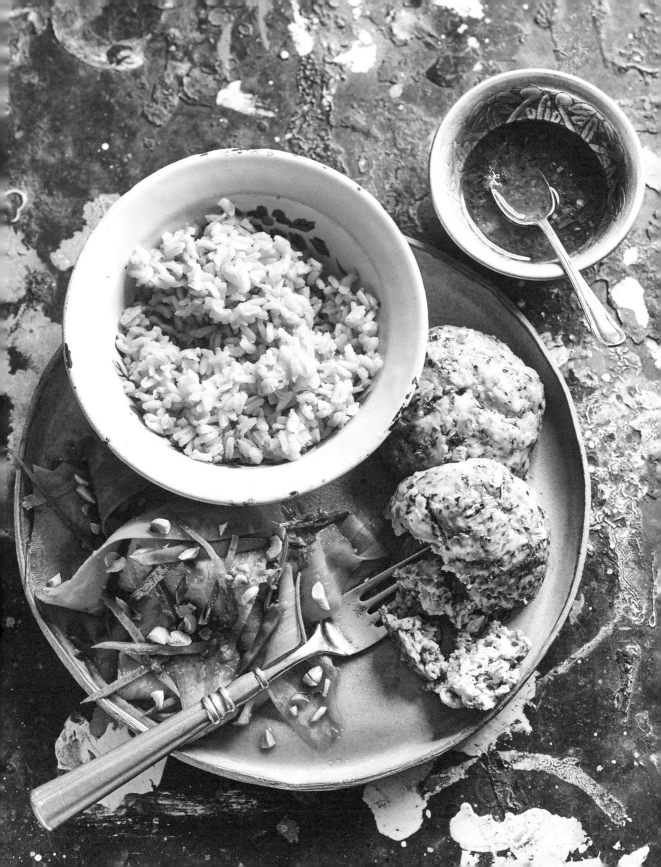

This is my perfect post-clinic meal. Even for someone who is as passionate about cooking as me, sometimes you just get home and can't be bothered to cook. This recipe solves that problem every time. Throw the ingredients in a roasting dish, prep a pesto and you have a gorgeous, fresh, nutrient-dense meal with leftovers for lunch the next day. It's simple, healthy and delicious.

Lazy Chickpea and Potato Roast with Pesto

serves 2

3 shallots, halved

400g tin chickpeas, drained and rinsed (or 200g dried chickpeas, cooked 'perfectly' – see page 96)

6 cherry tomatoes, halved (approximately 50g)

300g sweet potato, cut into 3cm cubes (unpeeled)

4 rosemary sprigs

4 thyme sprigs

1 fennel bulb, quartered

8 whole garlic cloves

3 tbsp extra-virgin olive oil

salt

For the pesto

15g basil leaves, roughly chopped

10g unsalted macadamia nuts (a small handful)

3 tbsp extra-virgin olive oil

5g Parmesan cheese, grated (optional)

Preheat the oven to 200°C/180°C fan/gas 6.

Put the shallots, chickpeas, tomatoes, sweet potato, rosemary, thyme, fennel and garlic in a roasting tray with a pinch of salt. Add the oil and toss to coat, then bake in the oven for 25 minutes.

To make the pesto, pound the basil, macadamia nuts and the soft pulp from three of the roasted garlic cloves in a pestle and mortar. Gradually drizzle in the oil, stirring constantly, until the pesto reaches your desired texture. Add the Parmesan (if using).

Serve the pesto on top of the warm roasted vegetables.

TIP

+ Add some roughly chopped spinach leaves for a burst of colour or some perfectly cooked cavolo nero (see page 102).

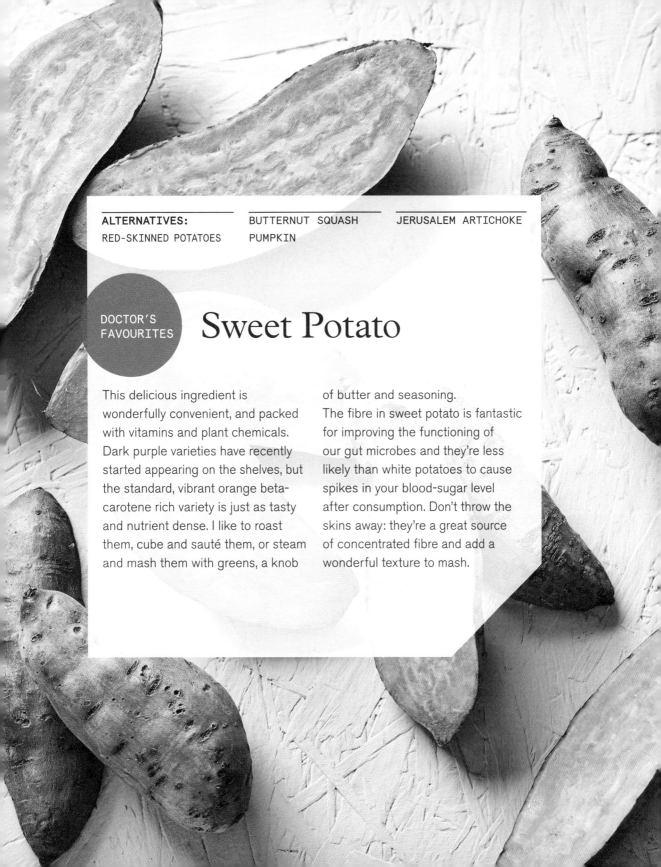

ALTERNATIVES:
RED-SKINNED POTATOES

BUTTERNUT SQUASH
PUMPKIN

JERUSALEM ARTICHOKE

DOCTOR'S FAVOURITES

Sweet Potato

This delicious ingredient is wonderfully convenient, and packed with vitamins and plant chemicals. Dark purple varieties have recently started appearing on the shelves, but the standard, vibrant orange beta-carotene rich variety is just as tasty and nutrient dense. I like to roast them, cube and sauté them, or steam and mash them with greens, a knob of butter and seasoning.

The fibre in sweet potato is fantastic for improving the functioning of our gut microbes and they're less likely than white potatoes to cause spikes in your blood-sugar level after consumption. Don't throw the skins away: they're a great source of concentrated fibre and add a wonderful texture to mash.

One of my best friends from university is now a highly qualified anaesthetist, but she's a hopeless cook! Despite growing up in Iran with a wealth of culinary heritage, she still hasn't learnt the kitchen basics, but even she can cook this meal. Sumac, a spice high in antioxidants, is used frequently in Persian cuisine. Tahini is a great source of calcium and B vitamins, and makes an appearance in both savoury and sweet dishes. I don't often use dried fruit in savoury meals, but in this dish it works very well.

Persian Chicken Thighs with Roasted Carrots and Tahini Yoghurt

serves 2

3 tbsp extra-virgin olive oil, plus extra for drizzling

1 tsp ground cinnamon

1 tsp sumac, plus extra for sprinkling

½ tsp chilli powder

4 bone-in, skin-on chicken thighs (or remove the skin if you prefer)

200g carrots, halved lengthways (unpeeled)

1 red onion, thinly sliced

5 garlic cloves, finely chopped

2–3 dried apricots, finely chopped

50ml water

10g unsalted, toasted pistachios, roughly ground

10g pine nuts, toasted

sea salt and freshly ground black pepper

red rice 'perfectly' cooked with a pinch of saffron (see page 99), to serve

For the tahini yoghurt

200g Greek yoghurt

3 tbsp tahini

grated zest and juice of ½ lemon

Mix 1 tablespoon of the oil with the cinnamon, sumac, chilli powder, and the seasoning in a large bowl. Add the chicken thighs, coat them in the mixture and leave to marinate in the fridge for at least 20 minutes (ideally overnight).

Preheat the oven to 200°C/180°C fan/gas 6.

Toss the carrots in a baking tray with 1 tablespoon of the oil and some seasoning and bake for 20 minutes, until soft and lightly browned.

Meanwhile, heat the remaining tablespoon of oil in an ovenproof frying pan over a low heat, add the onion, garlic and dried apricots and sauté for 2 minutes.

Place the marinated chicken thighs in the frying pan skin-side down and cook gently for about 6 minutes. Press the thighs to encourage the skin to colour and crisp up, then turn them over and cook for a further 2 minutes. Transfer to the oven for 12 minutes, or until the chicken is completely cooked through (if you don't have an ovenproof frying pan, just transfer the chicken to a baking tray).

Combine the tahini yoghurt ingredients in a bowl and sprinkle a little extra sumac on top.

Serve the chicken sprinkled with the toasted pistachios and pine nuts, with the yoghurt and roasted carrots alongside.

Mains

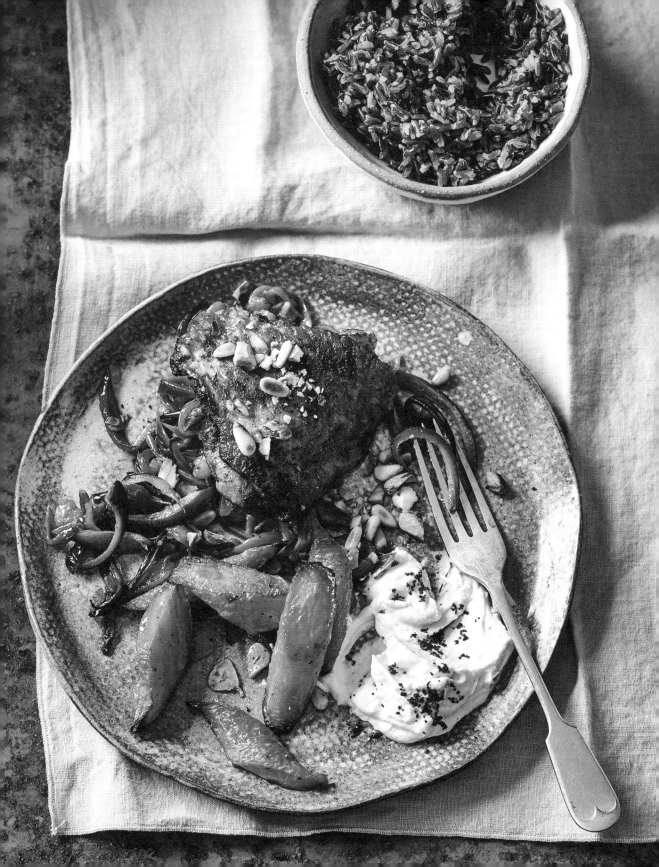

What I love about Italian cuisine is its simplicity and bold flavours. Anyone can make this beautiful, herby comfort meal in minutes. I use legumes that are full of fibre and associated with a reduced risk of multiple cancers. A core feature of the Mediterranean diet, legumes add a lot of substance to a meal and rosemary is a perfect match for the mushrooms and hazelnuts.

Italian Yellow Peas with Chestnut Mushrooms and Cavolo Nero

serves 2
with leftovers

3 tsp butter or extra-virgin olive oil

4 garlic cloves, roughly chopped

5 sun-dried tomatoes (dry, not in oil, if possible), roughly chopped

200g split yellow peas, soaked in water for 30 minutes (see page 96), then drained

1 tsp tomato paste

400ml boiling water

leaves from 2 rosemary sprigs

100g chestnut mushrooms, finely chopped

50g toasted hazelnuts, roughly crushed

80g cavolo nero, tough stems removed and leaves roughly chopped

sea salt and freshly ground black pepper

Heat 1 teaspoon of the butter or oil in a saucepan over a medium heat, add the garlic and sun-dried tomatoes, season with salt and pepper and sauté for 2 minutes. Add the soaked peas and tomato paste and cook for 2 minutes, stirring, then pour in the boiling water, cover, and cook for 25 minutes until soft and tender (most of the water will be absorbed).

Heat the remaining butter or oil in a frying pan over a medium heat. Add the rosemary, mushrooms and crushed hazelnuts and cook for 2 minutes, until the mushrooms are soft and lightly browned. Toss in the cavolo nero, stir for 1 minute, then add a splash of water, cover and let the greens lightly steam for 2 minutes.

Serve the greens on a platter topped with the yellow peas.

TIP

+ Add a drizzle of truffle oil if you want a luxurious twist. It marries well with the crunchy hazelnuts.

Using the fiery Jerk Paste you've made (see page 249) or bought, get ready for some sweet and chilli contrasts that will keep your taste buds guessing. Butternut squash is source of vitamin A and the sweet flesh is a lovely accompaniment to the highly spiced Jamaican spice blend. Since working at the community kitchen 'Made in Hackney' I've been more mindful of food wastage: cooking the butternut squash skin is a really cool way of using part of the veg I would otherwise bin. If you can't get hold of plantain, unripe bananas work well.

Jerk Squash and Celeriac with Plantain

serves 4

3 tbsp coconut oil, plus extra for the squash skins and plantain

300g butternut squash, peeled and cut into 2cm cubes (keep the skin strips)

1 plantain (about 150g), cut diagonally into 1cm slices

2 large tomatoes, roughly chopped

2 spring onions, roughly chopped

2 tsp tomato paste

grated zest and juice of 1 lime

300g celeriac, peeled and cut into 2cm cubes

2 tsp Jerk Paste (see page 249, or shop-bought)

2 tsp coconut cream

300ml vegetable stock or water

20g coriander, leaves and stalks finely chopped

sea salt and freshly ground black pepper

Preheat the oven to 180°C/160°C fan/gas 4.

Coat the pieces of butternut skin and plantain with coconut oil, spread them out on a baking tray, season with salt and pepper and bake in the oven for 15 minutes until the butternut squash skin is crispy and the plantain browned.

Meanwhile, melt 1 tablespoon of the coconut oil in a large saucepan over a medium heat. Add the tomatoes and spring onions and cook for 2 minutes, then transfer to a blender or food processor with the tomato paste and lime juice and zest. Blitz to form a purée.

Heat the remaining coconut oil in the same saucepan, add the butternut squash and celeriac, season with salt and pepper and sauté for 4–5 minutes until coloured. Add the jerk paste, coconut cream and tomato and lime purée and cook for 1 minute, stirring, then add the stock (or water) and coriander stalks and simmer for 15 minutes.

Serve the jerk squash and celeriac in bowls and garnish with the crispy butternut squash skins, coriander leaves and plantain.

TIP

+ There are plenty of carbohydrates in this dish so don't be tempted to serve it with a large portion of rice. Some vibrant greens or sweetcorn folded through the dish will do brilliantly.

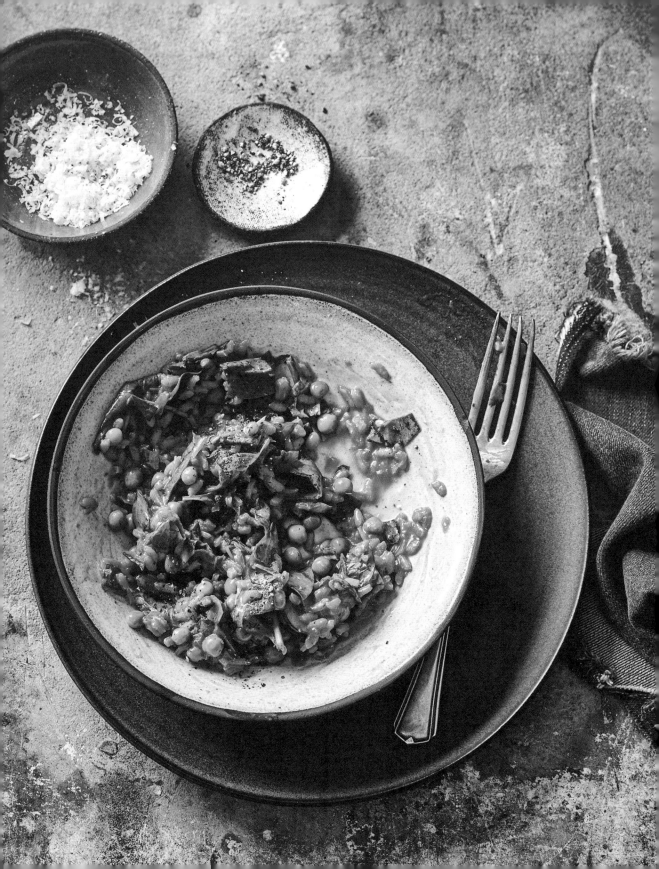

This is probably the most unlikely recipe you'll find in a 'healthy' cookbook – few healthy food bloggers dare use a 'nasty' refined rice like Arborio. However, I think we should really enjoy our food, and risotto is one of the most beautiful exports of Italian cooking. I've tried using different rice varieties like brown and wild rice to make risotto but they simply do not work! The process of cooking this meal – watching the pan and gradually adding stock, gently agitating the mixture and watching it transform into a creamy pan of deliciousness – makes you feel like a real home chef. The fats and starchy carbohydrate combination isn't ideal, but beetroot, peas and greens lighten up this otherwise dense meal.

Pea and Beetroot Risotto

serves 2

500ml vegetable stock

50g beetroot, grated

3 tbsp extra-virgin olive oil

2 shallots, finely diced

3 garlic cloves, finely diced

50g fresh porcini mushrooms, thinly sliced (or dried wild mushrooms, rehydrated)

leaves from 4 thyme sprigs

100g Arborio rice

30–40ml red wine (optional)

1 tsp butter

1 tsp grated Parmesan cheese

50g garden peas (fresh or thawed)

50g spinach, roughly chopped

sea salt and freshly ground black pepper

Put the stock in a saucepan with the beetroot, warm it through and keep it on the hob next to the saucepan you're going to cook the rice in.

Heat the oil in a saucepan over a medium heat, add the shallots, garlic, mushrooms and thyme, season with salt and pepper and sauté for 2–3 minutes to make the 'sofrito'. Add the rice and toast it in the oil for 2–3 minutes, then splash in the red wine (if using) and allow it to be absorbed by the rice.

Add one ladleful of the hot stock at a time and stir until it has been absorbed. Continue adding a little of the stock every 50–60 seconds, gently moving the rice around the pan. Once all the stock is absorbed (after 16–18 minutes), remove the pan from the heat and stir in the butter, cheese and peas. Cover the pan and set it aside for 1 minute, then remove the lid and fold the spinach through the mixture until wilted.

TIPS

+ You can use small brown mushrooms if you can't find porcini.
+ I serve this with steamed beans or broccoli, so you can still experience the risotto's amazing flavours without the heaviness.

ALTERNATIVES: GOLDEN BEETROOT   RAINBOW CHARD
RADISH   CHARD   RADICCHIO

DOCTOR'S FAVOURITES

Beetroot

This cheap, vibrant vegetable is known to improve protection against cardiovascular disease, as well as enhance athletic performance because of its ability to increase levels of nitric oxide in the blood. There is also some evidence to suggest that it may have a role in reducing atherosclerosis and treating high blood pressure, as well as the potential for preventing cognitive decline. Its robust, earthy flavour stands up well to roasting and I like to mix it up by finely slicing it raw into sautéed vegetables with cumin. I try to eat it a few times a week, as it is one of the most phytochemical-rich vegetables and one of the richest sources of anthocyanins that we have access to in this country. Purple sweet potato, goji berries and pomegranate are all touted for their health benefits, but common beetroot is just as impressive. Eat it whole, as its fibre content is fantastic and lost by juicing.

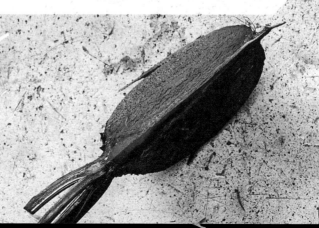

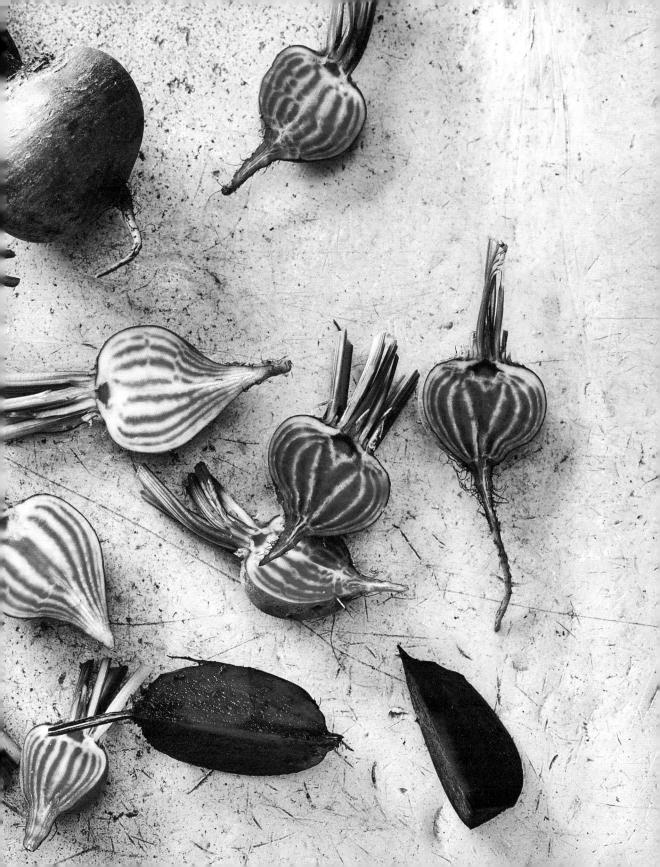

Summer signals the arrival of fresh, vibrant greens, gorgeous, earthy herbs and tons of produce to experiment with. My favourite summer ingredient is broad beans. They're cheap and widely available, and a rich source of protein and fibre. This meal with its polyphenol-rich dressing is just the ticket for a rapid light lunch.

serves 2
with leftovers

Summer Saluting Salad

For the platter

20g butter (or 3 tbsp olive oil)

3 spring onions, roughly chopped

5 sun-dried tomatoes in oil (or dried tomatoes rehydrated in warm water for 5 minutes), roughly chopped

100g green beans, trimmed and roughly chopped

100g podded broad beans

1 pointed cabbage (about 200g), quartered

150ml vegetable or chicken stock

100g quinoa, cooked 'perfectly' (see page 100)

sea salt and freshly ground black pepper

10g flaked almonds, toasted, to serve

For the dressing

20ml extra-virgin olive oil

leaves from 4 thyme sprigs

leaves from 4 oregano sprigs

grated zest and juice of 1 lemon

Melt the butter in a large frying pan over a medium heat, add the spring onions, sun-dried tomatoes, green and broad beans, season with salt and pepper and cook for 4 minutes.

Add the cabbage to the pan cut-side down and let it brown for 1 minute. Pour in the stock, cover and cook for about 6 minutes (adding more stock or water if it completely dries out).

Mix the dressing ingredients in a bowl, then remove the vegetables from the heat and pour the dressing over them.

Serve with the quinoa, sprinkled with the toasted flaked almonds.

TIP

+ For a slight kick, add some dried chilli flakes to the pan when you add the broad beans.

I was raised in the Sikh faith and some of my earliest childhood memories are of our weekly visits to the local temple, listening to *shabads* (hymns) and taking in the distinctive smell of the communal eating hall, known as the langar. In every Sikh temple the world over, these kitchens have for centuries offered vegetarian food to people of any race or background, and still do. My early experiences in the temple, where food was treated with such respect, have shaped my understanding of its importance to life. These lentils are exceptionally nutritious, easy to make and absolutely delicious. I hope you enjoy the process of making the dish and think of how this meal is being prepared in the same way, every day, across the world.

Auspicious 'Langar' Lentils

serves 2

250g brown lentils, soaked for 8–10 hours, drained and rinsed

900ml vegetable stock or water

3 tsp butter, ghee or coconut oil

1 red onion, finely diced

1 green chilli, deseeded and finely chopped

8cm piece of root ginger, peeled and grated

½ tsp garam masala (see page 240 for my own blend), plus extra for serving

50g spinach, finely chopped

100g probiotic yoghurt

sea salt and freshly ground black pepper

100g cooked red wild rice (50g dried red wild rice, cooked 'perfectly' – see page 99 – or from a packet), to serve

For the Indian side salad

½ red onion, thinly sliced

1 green chilli, thinly sliced (not for the faint hearted)

10cm piece of cucumber, thinly sliced

juice of ½ lime

Put the soaked lentils in a saucepan, season with salt and pepper and add the stock or water. Bring to a simmer over a medium heat and cook for 45 minutes, or until the lentils are soft, then remove the pan from the heat.

Mash half the lentils in the saucepan (with a masher or stick blender) to give the dish a thicker, rustic consistency.

Melt the butter, ghee or coconut oil in a frying pan over a medium heat, add the onion, chilli, ginger and garam masala, season with salt and pepper and sauté for 2–3 minutes. Add the mixture to the lentils along with the spinach, stir it through and cover for 2 minutes to gently wilt the spinach before serving.

Combine the ingredients for the salad in a bowl, and put the yoghurt in a separate bowl, with a dash of garam masala.

Serve the lentils with the salad, yoghurt and rice.

TIP

+ For an indulgent twist, add a splash of cream to the lentils before serving.

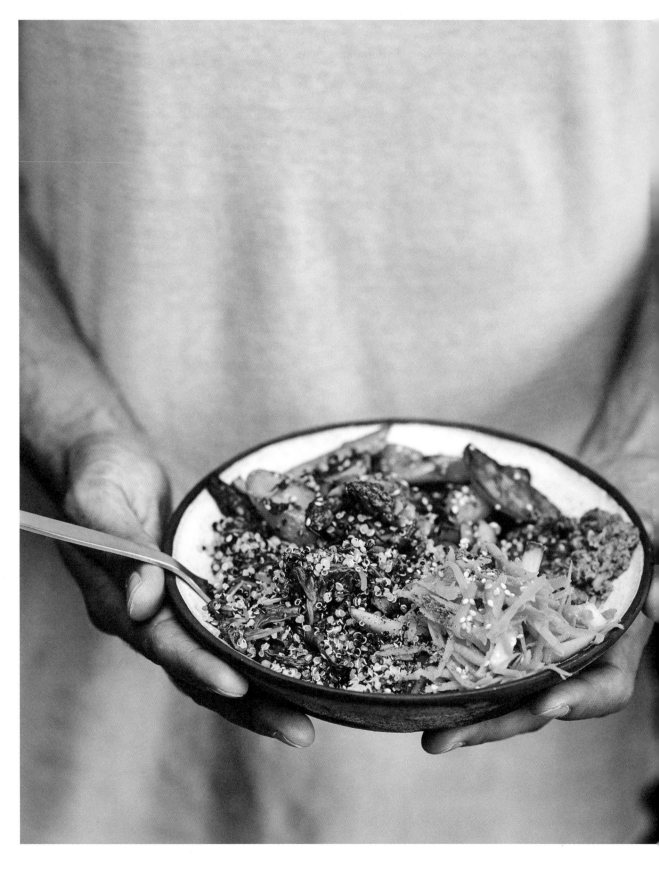

When patients ask me what they should be eating, I've got into the habit of pulling up images of 'Buddha bowls'. It's a striking visual representation of how I believe we should be trying to eat. They are a fantastic mixture of different coloured vegetables, wholegrains and spices and it's an easy visual for people to utilise at home. When you look at your plates I want you to count colours not calories. Making this sort of meal from scratch is super-simple, despite the long ingredients list. Play around with different root vegetables and use different spices – it's very easy when you know the basics.

serves 2
generously

Za'atar Bowl

4 carrots, 3 quartered lengthways and 1 grated

50g asparagus spears, trimmed

200g sweet potato, cut into thin chips (unpeeled)

4 tbsp extra-virgin olive oil

3 thyme sprigs

1 tsp cayenne pepper

150g cooked puy lentils (75g dried puy lentils, cooked 'perfectly' – see page 96 – or from a packet)

1 tbsp tahini

50ml water

1 garlic clove

100g spinach

2 tsp Za'atar Spice Blend (see page 242, or shop-bought), plus extra for sprinkling

150g cooked tricolour quinoa (100g dried quinoa, cooked ' perfectly' – see page 100 – or from a packet)

10cm piece of cucumber, cut into matchsticks (unpeeled)

sea salt and freshly ground black pepper

20g sesame seeds, toasted, to serve

Preheat the oven to 200°C/180°C fan/gas 6.

Put the quartered carrots, asparagus spears and sweet potato chips in a roasting tray, drizzle with 1 tablespoon of the oil, add the thyme and cayenne, season with salt and pepper and toss to coat. Roast in the oven for 25 minutes, until soft and lightly browned.

Meanwhile, put the lentils, tahini, water and garlic in a blender or food processor with a pinch of salt and pepper and blitz to form a hummus-like mixture.

Heat another tablespoon of the oil in a frying pan, add the spinach and za'atar and cook for 1 minute until wilted. Fold the spinach through the cooked quinoa (it can be warm or cold).

Mix the grated carrot and cucumber matchsticks in a bowl with another tablespoon of the oil.

Build your bowl (see opposite) and dress with the remaining oil, sprinkling it with more za'atar and toasted sesame seeds.

Parsley offers so many wonderful health benefits. I try to use this delicious herb on a weekly basis. The bitter taste is testament to its rich phytonutrient content. Making tabbouleh is a beautiful way of extracting all those plant chemicals while mellowing the strong taste of the herb. Hailing from the Middle East, tabbouleh is a wonderful marriage of ingredients easily found on British soil. Super-simple to prepare in bulk, I often take this in my Tupperware to work, especially when there isn't anywhere to warm up your food. I use quinoa as a protein-rich alternative to cracked wheat.

serves 2
with leftovers

Dukkah Chickpea Tabbouleh

400g tinned chickpeas, drained and rinsed (200g dried chickpeas, cooked 'perfectly' – see page 96)

3 tsp Egyptian dukkah

3 tbsp extra-virgin olive oil, plus extra for drizzling

1 white onion, finely diced

15g parsley, leaves and stalks finely chopped

15cm piece of cucumber, cubed (unpeeled)

150g cooked red quinoa (100g dried quinoa, cooked 'perfectly' – see page 100 – or from a packet)

100g broccoli sprouts (or pea shoots, watercress, or mung bean sprouts)

1 tsp dried chilli flakes

10g coriander, leaves and stalks chopped

Preheat the oven to 200°C/180°C fan/gas 6.

Put the chickpeas in a bowl with the dukkah and oil and toss to coat. Spread the chickpeas out on a baking tray and bake in the oven for 12 minutes, until firm and toasted.

Meanwhile, combine the onion, parsley, cucumber, quinoa, broccoli sprouts and chilli flakes in a bowl. Mix through the baked chickpeas while they're still warm and drizzle with plenty of extra-virgin olive oil.

Garnish with coriander and serve.

TIPS

+ Use za'atar (see page 242) instead of the dukkah for another herby twist on the classic dish.
+ If you're making the tabbouleh ahead of time, leave out the coriander until ready to serve, to avoid it going limp.

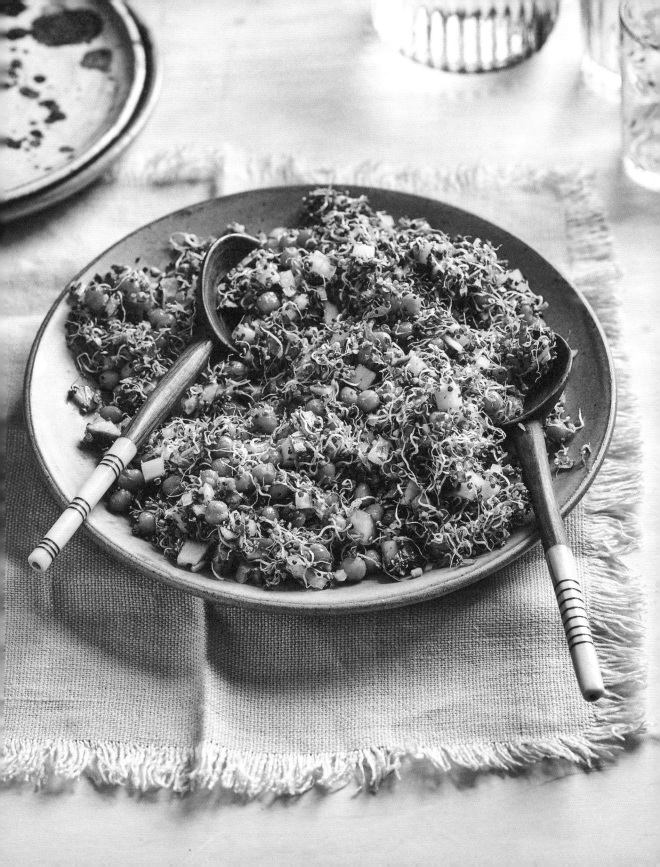

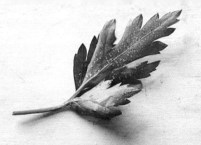

ALTERNATIVES:
CORIANDER

BASIL
OREGANO

ROSEMARY
SAGE

Parsley

Parsley has so many wonderful benefits. Its distinctive taste is testament to its rich quantity of beneficial plant chemicals called flavones, which are known for their potential role in dementia protection, as well as scavenging harmful chemicals from the blood. Parsley also contains vitamins like folate, essential for DNA repair and replication. In Ayurvedic and Eastern tradition, herbs like parsley, coriander and basil have long been recognised for their medicinal properties, and there is fascinating scientific evidence confirming these long-held beliefs. Tabbouleh is one of my favourite ways to serve parsley, but it works equally well chopped and mixed into mashed celeriac or folded into curries.

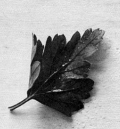
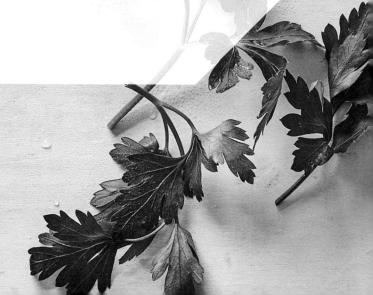

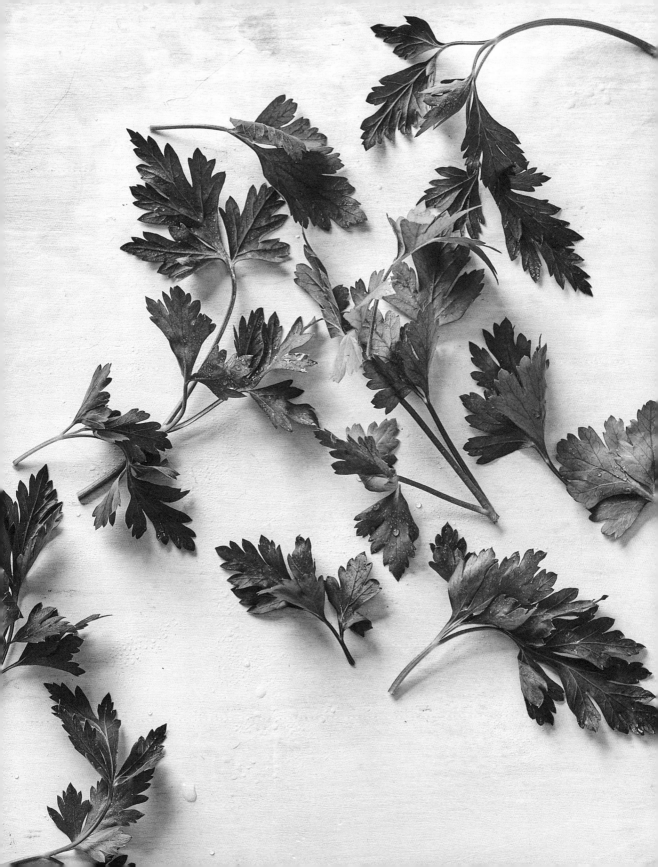

There are so many beautiful ingredients in this dish. The kofte are packed with nutty lentils, healthy-fat-rich extra-virgin olive oil and incredible polyphenol-rich herbs. Parsley, an often overlooked herb, has huge health benefits packed into each intensely flavoured leaf. This dish nods to elements of Mediterranean cuisine that make eating both pleasurable and healthy, and is a celebration of longevity-promoting Grecian flavours.

Greek Kofte with Tahini and Garlic Dip

serves 4

For the kofte

100g sweet potato, grated (unpeeled)

50g coriander, leaves and stalks roughly chopped

50g parsley, leaves and stalks roughly chopped

leaves from 4 mint sprigs, roughly chopped

4 garlic cloves, grated

½ tsp ground cumin

2 tbsp extra-virgin olive oil

100g full-fat Greek yoghurt

1 egg

200g cooked puy lentils (100g dried puy lentils, cooked 'perfectly' – see page 96 – or from a packet)

sea salt and freshly ground black pepper

For the tahini and garlic dip

2 tbsp tahini

100g full-fat Greek yoghurt

grated zest and juice of ½ lemon

1 garlic clove, grated

For the salad

50g Kalamata olives, pitted and halved

100g spinach, roughly chopped

25g parsley, leaves and stalks roughly chopped

150g cooked red, tricolour or white quinoa (100g dried quinoa, cooked 'perfectly' – see page 100 – or from a packet)

2 tbsp extra-virgin olive oil

Preheat the oven to 200°C/180°C fan/gas 6 and line a baking sheet with greaseproof paper.

Combine all the ingredients for the kofte in a large bowl and season. Put the mixture in a food processor and pulse until evenly blended but not smooth – you want to keep some texture. Spoon 8 large kofte shapes of the mixture onto the lined baking sheet and bake in the oven for 25 minutes until browned and crisp on the outside.

Meanwhile, mix the ingredients for the tahini and garlic dip together in a bowl and season to taste.

Combine the olives, spinach, parsley and cooked quinoa in a bowl and drizzle over the oil. Serve the kofte, dip and salad on a platter to share, and dig in.

TIP

+ Add a sprinkle of chilli powder to the dip to give it a spicy kick.

Mains

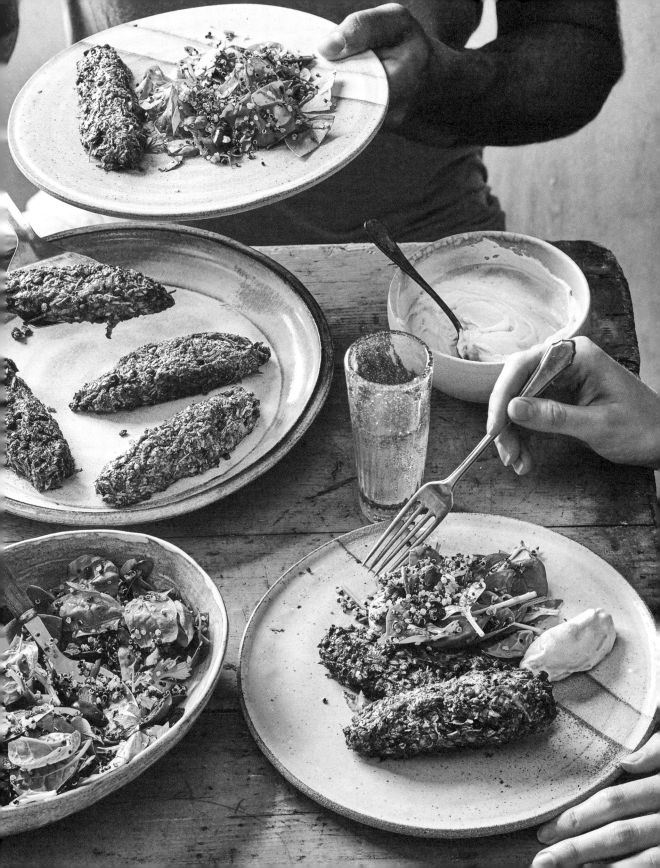

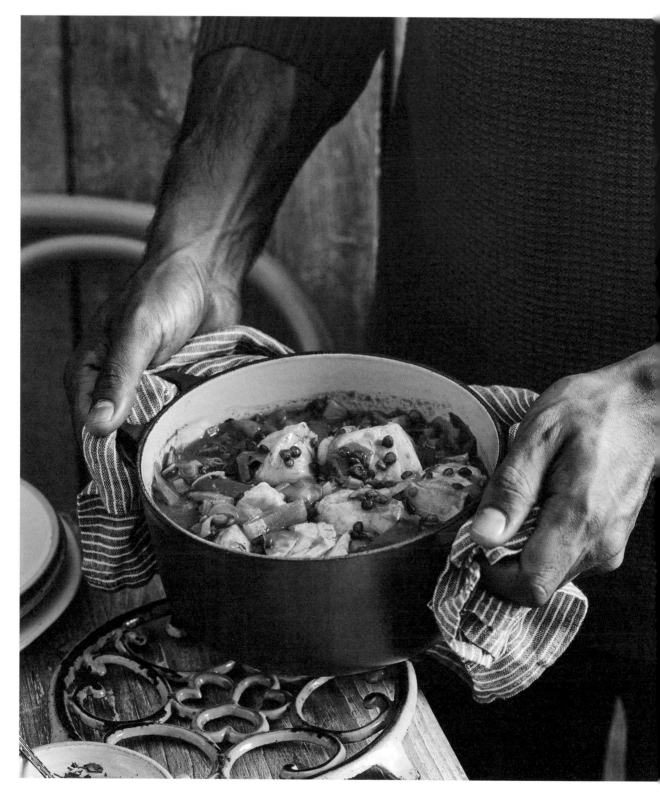

196   Mains

One-pot dishes are my favourite midweek meal. They're comforting and always provide leftovers for lunch. This speedy fish supper is a beautiful mix of Mediterranean spices and punchy flavours. Cooked tomatoes release a gorgeous sweetness and they're a source of lycopene, a phytochemical shown to potentially reduce the incidence of prostate cancer. A quick dressing using polyphenol-rich coriander and lemon brings a great kick of acidity to the sweetness of the red peppers and leek.

Mediterranean Cod One-Pot

serves 4

6 tbsp extra-virgin olive oil

2 shallots, roughly chopped

4 garlic cloves, finely chopped

3 large tomatoes, roughly chopped

1 romano red pepper, deseeded and roughly chopped

15g coriander, leaves and stalks roughly chopped

400g leeks, washed, trimmed and roughly chopped

1 tsp sweet paprika

1 tsp chilli powder

300ml vegetable or chicken stock

300g cooked puy lentils (200g dried puy lentils, cooked 'perfectly' – see page 96 – or from a packet)

400g boneless, skinless cod fillets

½ tbsp dried chilli flakes

grated zest and juice of ½ lemon

sea salt and freshly ground black pepper

Heat 3 tablespoons of the oil in a saucepan over a medium heat, add the shallots and garlic and sauté for a few minutes until soft. Add the tomatoes, red pepper, coriander stalks, leeks, sweet paprika and chilli powder, season with salt and pepper and cook, stirring, for 2 minutes.

Pour in the stock and puy lentils and bring to a simmer for 5 minutes. Add the cod, cover and cook for a further 8 minutes, until the fish is cooked through.

Mix the remaining oil in a bowl with the chilli flakes and coriander leaves, then stir in the lemon zest and juice.

Serve the stew in large bowls with the dressing drizzled on top.

TIPS

+ Try using other legumes in place of the lentils, such as white beans, chickpeas or kidney beans.
+ Play around with different spices: harissa or chipotle both work well.

The sweet, spicy sauce of patatas bravas is unmistakeable. My favourite memory of eating this traditional tapas dish was people-watching at a food market eatery in Barcelona. I'm so fond of Spanish food and it can make a healthy and super-quick midweek meal. Cooking the fish enclosed in paper means you can't go wrong: it's such a simple method. Celeriac and turnip are fantastic root vegetables with great fibre content, and are an ideal substitute for potatoes with the bravas sauce.

Fish in a Paper Bag with Celeriac Bravas

serves 2

2 tbsp extra-virgin olive oil

200g peeled celeriac, cut into
    2cm cubes

200g turnip, cut into 2cm
    cubes (unpeeled)

50g radicchio, finely chopped

100g cherry tomatoes,
    roughly chopped

sea salt and freshly ground
    black pepper

For the fish in a bag

1 carrot, peeled lengthways into
    thin strips with a vegetable peeler

½ red pepper, thickly sliced

1 tbsp extra-virgin olive oil

4 thyme sprigs

4 oregano sprigs

200g boneless, skinless cod fillet

For the spicy bravas sauce

1 tbsp extra-virgin olive oil

1 garlic clove, finely chopped

200ml passata

1 tsp tomato paste

1 tsp dried chilli flakes

1 tsp sweet paprika

10g parsley, leaves and stalks
    finely chopped

Preheat the oven to 200°C/180°C fan/gas 6.

Start by preparing the fish in a bag. Put the carrot, red pepper, olive oil, thyme and oregano on a large sheet of baking parchment. Place the fish on top and season with salt and pepper. Seal the package tightly by crimping the edges of the paper together over the fish, pop it on a baking tray and bake in the oven for 8 minutes.

Meanwhile, heat the 2 tablespoons of oil in a frying pan, add the celeriac and turnip, season with salt and pepper and sauté for 8 minutes until lightly coloured and cooked through. Transfer to a bowl, add the radicchio and tomatoes and toss to combine.

To make the spicy bravas sauce, heat the oil in a saucepan, add the garlic and fry until browned but not burnt. Add the passata, tomato paste, chilli flakes and paprika, heat through, then fold in the parsley.

Cover the celeriac and turnips with the bravas sauce. Unwrap the fish as soon as you take it out of the oven and serve it with the celeriac bravas.

TIPS
+ Feel free to swap the cod for haddock, pollock or mackerel fillets.
+ You can swap the sharp, beautifully coloured radicchio for
    other nutrient-dense greens if you prefer, such as rocket.

Mains

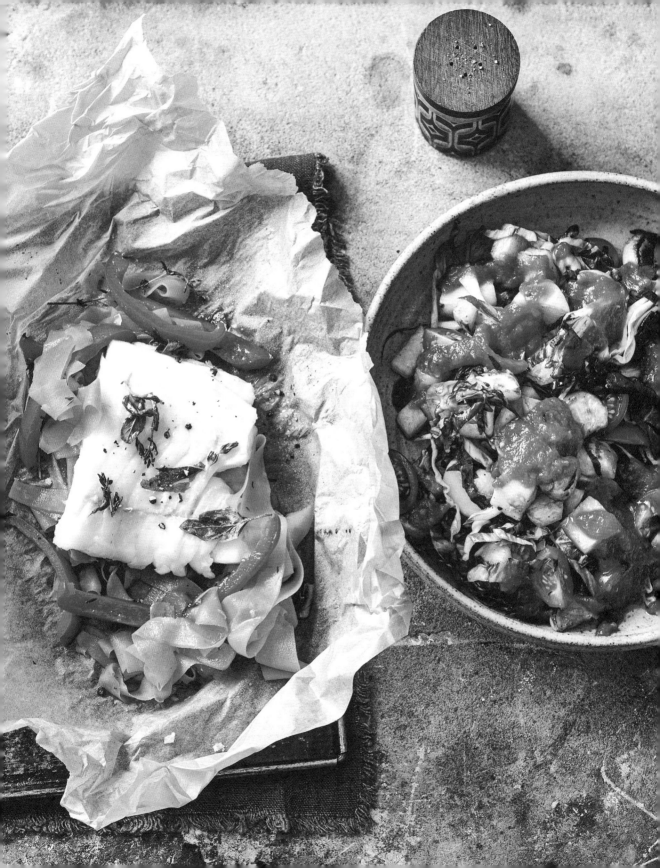

This is perhaps the most important dish I ever cooked. It was the first recipe I was taught by my mother before I went to university. I remember thinking how effortless she made it look and how simple it was to copy. From week one my reputation for being 'the cook' at university was set. While everyone else was adding ready-made Bolognese sauce to their overcooked pasta, I was imbuing the student halls of residence with the scent of Thai basil and coconut. This curry has a beautiful mix of exotic spices and a creamy texture. Lemongrass has been shown to have anti-cancer effects in some small studies, but the main reason I use it is because it adds a delicate citrus edge to this elegant curry.

serves 4

Lemongrass Thai Curry

2 tbsp coconut oil

1 shallot, diced

1 stick of lemongrass, bruised

thumb-sized piece of galangal or ginger, peeled and grated

3 garlic cloves, finely chopped

500g skinless chicken breast or firm tofu, cut into 4cm-thick slices or cubes

400g tin coconut milk (or 2 tbsp coconut cream mixed with 300ml hot water)

3 kaffir lime leaves (optional)

1 red chilli, split lengthways and deseeded (leave the seeds in if you like it hot)

2 tsp fish sauce (optional)

leaves from 3 Thai basil or regular basil sprigs, roughly chopped

2 tbsp soy sauce

200g pak choy (or any dark green leafy vegetable), roughly chopped

¼ head red cabbage, shredded

300g cooked black or red rice (200g dried rice, cooked 'perfectly' – see pages 99–100 – or from a packet)

Melt the coconut oil in a saucepan over a medium heat, add the shallot, lemongrass, galangal or ginger and the garlic and sauté for a few minutes until the shallot has softened. Add the chicken or tofu to the pan and sauté for a further 4 minutes until browned.

Add the coconut milk (or cream and hot water) to the pan along with the kaffir lime leaves (if using), red chilli, fish sauce (if using), basil and soy sauce and simmer for 11–12 minutes, then add the pak choy and cook for a further 2 minutes.

Fold the red cabbage through the cooked rice and serve it with the curry in bowls.

TIPS
+ Add a heaped teaspoon of peanut butter with the coconut milk to make it even more luxurious and creamy.
+ Scatter with crushed peanuts and garnish with chilli.

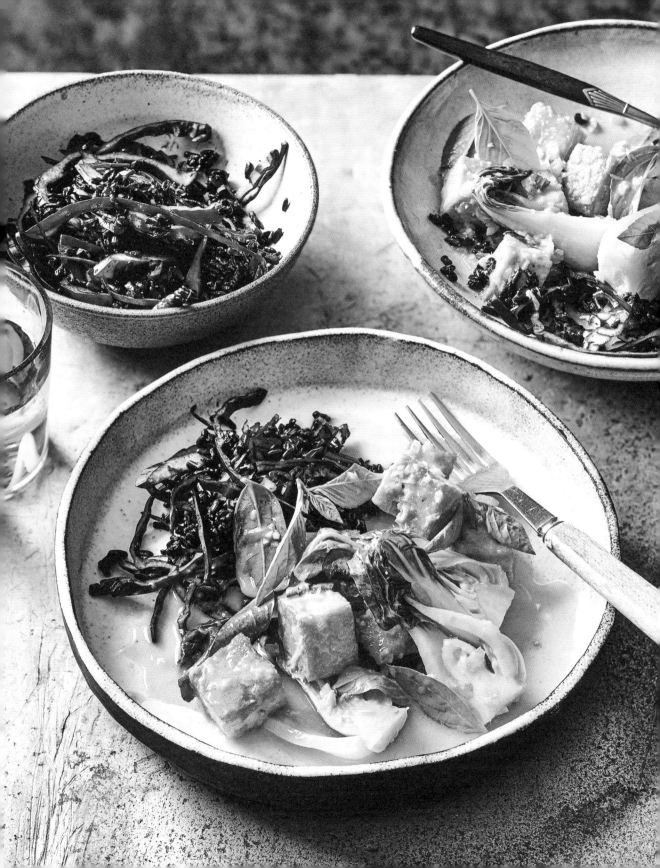

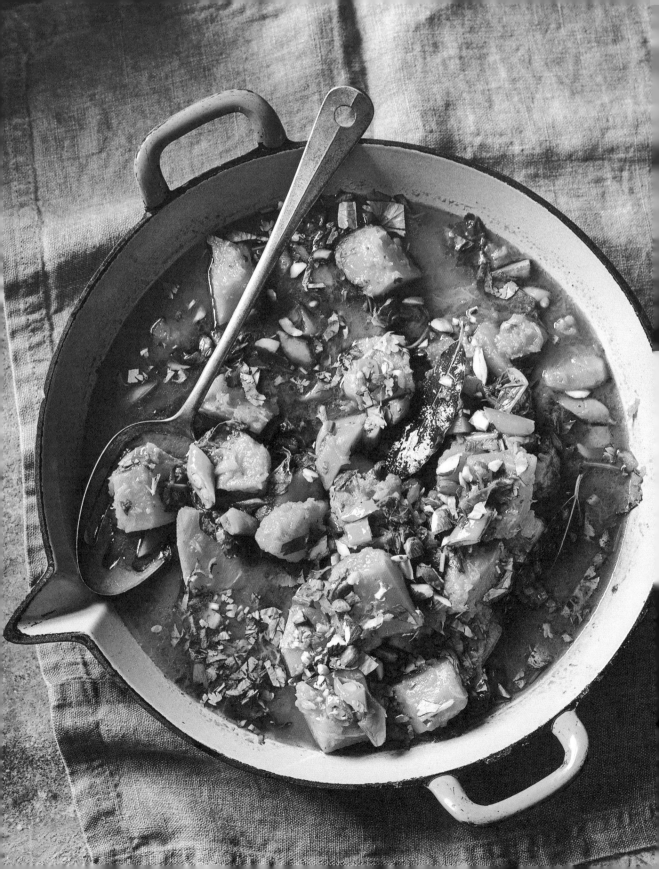

Flavour-packed, slow-cooked dishes are the simplest yet most satisfying and comforting meals. This rich Massaman curry can be made with meat, but I love using butternut squash instead. It takes on the spices really well and, with the extra veg, the dish has plenty of micronutrients. Greens, squash and other yellow/orange coloured vegetables are dense sources of pro-vitamin A and offer vital phytonutrients for immunity and eye health. This recipe makes enough for lunch the next day (to make your co-workers envious).

serves 4

Butternut Massaman Curry

2 tbsp coconut oil

3 tsp Massaman Paste (see page 248) or shop-bought paste

100g coconut cream

500g butternut squash, peeled, deseeded and cut into 4cm cubes

300ml vegetable stock or water

2 tsp fish sauce (optional)

2 bay leaves

1 tsp runny honey

50g sugar snap peas, roughly chopped

50g spinach, roughly chopped

25g coriander leaves, roughly chopped

20g dry roasted almonds, roughly crushed

sea salt and freshly ground black pepper

cooked brown rice, to serve (optional)

Melt the coconut oil in a saucepan over a medium heat, add the Massaman paste and fry for 1 minute, then stir in the coconut cream. Add the cubed butternut squash, season with salt and pepper and cook, stirring, for 2–3 minutes, until lightly coloured.

Pour in the stock or water, add the fish sauce (if using), bay leaves and honey, cover and simmer for 25 minutes, until the vegetables are soft and the sauce has reduced.

Remove from the heat, fold in the sugar snap peas and spinach and cover for 2 minutes. The heat of the curry will lightly cook them.

Garnish the curry with the coriander and crushed almonds and serve it on its own or with a little brown rice on the side to soak up the creamy sauce.

TIPS

+ Use soy sauce instead of fish sauce, if you wish.
+ Add coconut milk with the stock to make the curry sauce extra creamy.

A perfect match for my sister's Marinara Sauce (page 144), my 'meat' balls are made with puy lentils, wild mushrooms and flaxseeds – you will not miss the red meat! I tend to prepare a big batch of these because they disappear quickly. Packed with beautiful Italian herbs and spices, they will imbue your kitchen with Mediterranean vibes. The Mediterranean diet is universally one of the most researched diets proven to reduce the incidence of cancer, diabetes and heart disease and, contrary to popular belief, it actually features little meat. Experiment with different herbs and find what works for you.

serves 4

Meatless Meatballs

3 tbsp extra-virgin olive oil

5 garlic cloves, crushed

200g fresh porcini mushrooms (or wild or chestnut), finely chopped

leaves from 2 rosemary sprigs, finely chopped

6 sun-dried tomatoes in oil, finely chopped

1 tsp dried chilli flakes

500g cooked puy lentils (250g dried puy lentils, cooked 'perfectly' – see page 96 – or from a packet)

3 tbsp ground flaxseeds

300g wholegrain or black bean fettucine

2 carrots, peeled lengthways into thin strips with a vegetable peeler

500ml Jasmin's Marinara Sauce (see page 144), warmed through

Preheat the oven to 200°C/180°C fan/gas 6 and line a baking tray with baking parchment.

Heat the oil in a frying pan over a medium heat, add the garlic, mushrooms, rosemary, sun-dried tomatoes and chilli flakes and sauté for 2–3 minutes, until the mushrooms have softened. Stir in the lentils, then transfer the mixture to a blender or food processor with the flaxseed and blitz for just long enough to combine everything and until all the ingredients have a uniform texture. Form the mixture into 16 balls.

Put the balls on the lined baking tray and bake in the oven for 20 minutes, until crisp on the outside and hot through.

Meanwhile, cook the fettucine in a pan of boiling water for 6 minutes (or according to the packet instructions), throwing in the carrot strips for the last minute of cooking time to soften them.

Drain the fettucine and carrots and serve with the baked meatless meatballs and Marina Sauce.

TIP

+ If you're short of time you can easily serve this with some store-bought Italian tomato sauce with a few basil leaves thrown in for flavour.

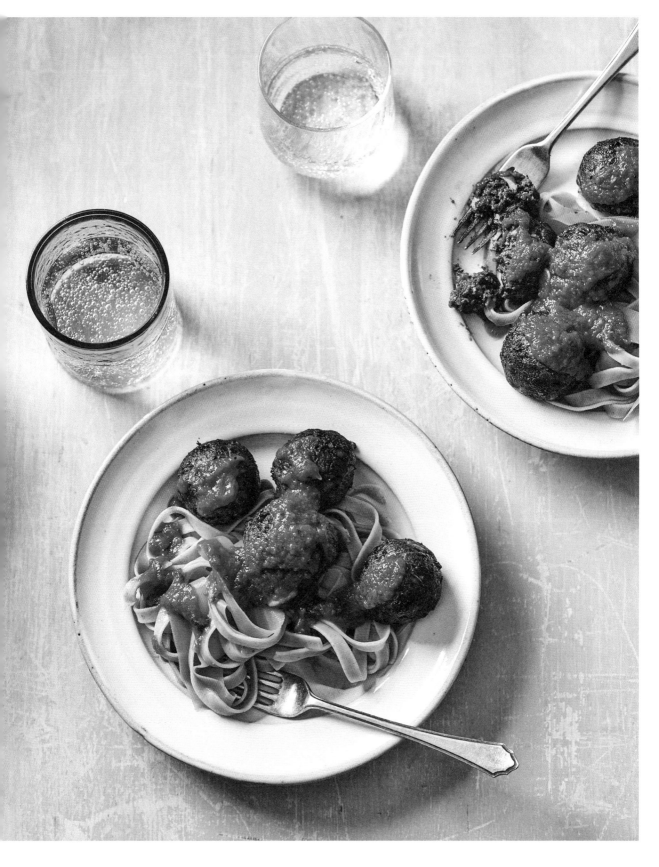

A source of fibre, phytonutrients and plant-based protein, there is so much nutrition in the humble pea. We use them a lot in Punjabi cuisine. The wealth of spices in this dish completely transforms plain frozen peas, and I hope you'll never look at them the same way again. I usually eat it with red rice and plain yoghurt or a side salad.

serves 2
with leftovers

Punjabi Matar

2 tbsp coconut oil

1 tsp coriander seeds, lightly bruised in a pestle and mortar

1 tsp cumin seeds, lightly bruised in a pestle and mortar

½ white onion, diced

300g peas (fresh or thawed)

½ tsp dried chilli flakes

150g tinned chopped tomatoes

50g spinach, finely chopped

sea salt and freshly ground black pepper

200g cooked red rice, (100g dried red rice – cooked 'perfectly' – see page 99), to serve

Melt the oil in a frying pan over a medium heat, add the spices and a pinch of salt and pepper and fry for 1 minute until fragrant. Then add the diced onion and cook for 2 minutes until lightly browned.

Add the peas and chilli flakes, then tip in the tomatoes. Bring to a simmer and cook for 3 minutes. Fold in the spinach, remove from the heat and cover for 2 minutes. Serve with the fragrant rice.

TIP

+ If you're preparing the rice from scratch, try adding a bay leaf, 2 cardamom pods and 1 cinnamon stick to the cooking water. It will create a wonderful spiced rice for the peas.

Most Indians will be surprised to see such a traditional dish in a modern cookbook, but when the classic is as perfect as this, I'm not going to mess around with it much. I remember as a teenager my parents told me that the spices in daal protected my tummy. I wasn't having any of it. That was until I started reading about clinical research examining the digestive effects of Indian spices such as clove, cumin and cardamom. Yet another 'I-told-you-so' moment. Yellow lentils are one of the easiest pulses to prepare from scratch, and this is one of the most nourishing recipes in my book. 'Tarka' is the name for flavoured, spiced oil.

serves 2

Tarka Daal

100g yellow lentils, soaked for 20 minutes (see page 96) and rinsed well

1 tsp turmeric

1 star anise

200ml water

25g spinach, thinly sliced

2 tbsp coconut oil

1 tsp black mustard seeds

1 tsp cumin seeds

2 cloves

1 cinnamon stick, broken in half

2 green cardamom pods

2 spring onions, thinly sliced

3 garlic cloves, finely chopped

3cm piece of root ginger, peeled and grated

5 cherry tomatoes, halved

juice of ½ lime

sea salt and freshly ground black pepper

Put the lentils in a pan with the turmeric, star anise and water, bring to a simmer over a medium heat and cook for 20 minutes until the lentils are soft and breaking apart. Take off the heat and, using a masher, roughly mash the lentils in the pan to create a gorgeous, creamy texture. Fold the spinach through the lentils and cover (the residual heat will lightly wilt the leaves).

Meanwhile, melt the coconut oil in a frying pan over a medium heat, add the mustard seeds, cumin seeds, cloves, cinnamon and cardamom and fry for 1–2 minutes until the mustard seeds begin to pop and the spices are fragrant. Add the spring onions, garlic, ginger and season with salt and pepper and sauté for 2–3 minutes until lightly browned. Add the tomatoes and let them soften a little. Remove the pan from the heat.

Mix half the 'tarka' through the lentils, divide the lentils between two bowls and spoon the rest of the tarka on top. Drizzle with the lime juice and serve.

TIPS
+ Don't worry about the mustard seeds if you can't find any.
+ Add a finely sliced green chilli with the ginger and garlic if you like a bit of heat.

Mains

Sometimes you just need the right flavours and ingredients thrown into a roasting dish and something magical happens. The hot and tangy combination of lime, chilli and turmeric is brilliant with cauliflower – the punchy, bold flavours heighten the enjoyment of this fantastic brassica vegetable. This is a favourite of mine to rustle up quickly after work. I like to add prawns, but poached chicken or white fish work well, too. I always make plenty, so there are leftovers to put in my Tupperware for the next day (the flavours intensify overnight).

Spiced Lime Cauliflower and Sweet Potato Bake with Prawns

serves 2
with leftovers

½ tsp turmeric

1 tsp chilli powder

5cm piece of root ginger, peeled and grated

6 tbsp extra-virgin olive oil

2 limes, halved

2 shallots, quartered lengthways and peeled

300g cauliflower, broken into florets

300g sweet potato, cut lengthways into 2–3cm-thick wedges

250g raw shelled jumbo prawns, deveined

100g spinach, finely chopped

sea salt and freshly ground black pepper

Preheat the oven to 200°C/180°C fan/gas 6.

Mix the spices, ginger and 5 tablespoons of the olive oil in a bowl and season with salt and pepper. Squeeze in the juice from the limes.

Finely chop the juiced lime halves. Spread them out in a baking tray with the shallots, cauliflower florets and sweet potato. Drizzle over the spiced oil and coat the ingredients well, then bake in the oven for 35 minutes, stirring halfway through to ensure they cook evenly.

After the vegetables have been in the oven for 30 minutes, heat the remaining oil in a frying pan over a medium heat. Add the prawns, season with salt and pepper and sauté for 2 minutes, then turn them over and sauté for a further minute, or until cooked through. Remove from the heat, add the spinach, stir and cover the pan for 1–2 minutes – the residual heat will wilt the spinach.

Transfer the tangy baked cauliflower and sweet potato to a serving dish, fold in the prawns and spinach and dress it with the oil from the baking tray.

Mains

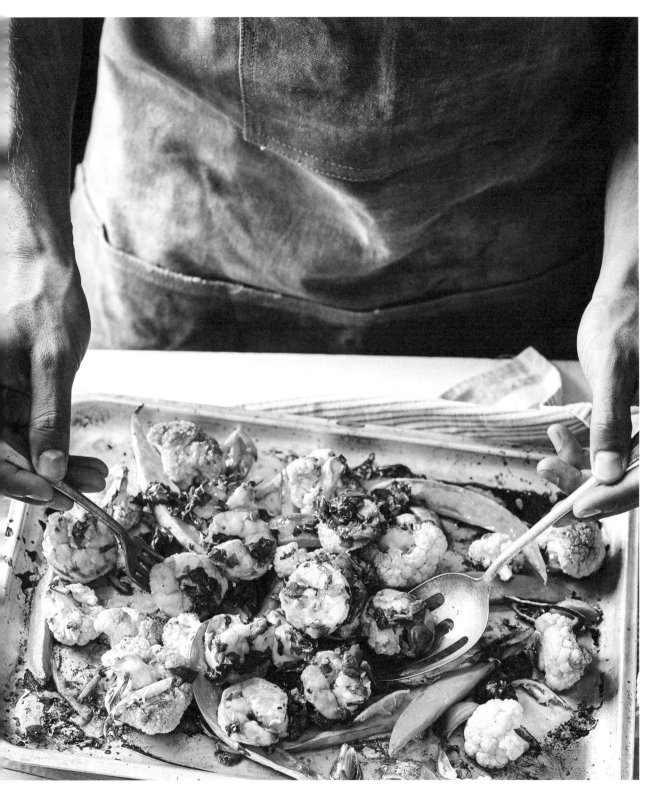

Fresh fish doesn't have a pungent odour and it is one of the simplest things to cook. This meal takes no time at all and sometimes I eat it straight out of the pan. I add a mixture of fresh, colourful chard and pak choy containing plant compounds called glucosinolates, known for their ability to prevent cancer and samphire is a mineral-rich marine plant that grows all over the British Isles. We need to make more use of these nutrient-dense and widely available foods!

One-pan Haddock with Mushrooms and Lemony Greens

serves 2

3 tbsp extra-virgin olive oil

2 garlic cloves, chopped

50g chestnut mushrooms, finely chopped

150g pak choy, roughly chopped

50g samphire (optional)

100g rainbow chard, roughly chopped

100ml boiling water

300g boneless, skinless haddock fillet (cod, pollock or salmon also work well)

grated zest and juice of 1 lemon

½ tsp cayenne pepper

sea salt and freshly ground black pepper

Heat 2 tablespoons of the oil in a large frying pan over a low–medium heat, add the garlic and mushrooms, season with salt and pepper and sauté for 2 minutes.

Toss in the greens and colourful chard and cook for 2 minutes. Gently pour the boiling water around the edge of the pan. Place the fish fillet on top of the vegetables, cover and cook for 7–8 minutes (adding a touch more boiling water if the 100ml water evaporates before the fish is cooked), until the fish is cooked through and flakes easily when gently prodded with a fork.

Remove the fish and vegetables from the pan and deglaze the pan over the heat with the lemon juice, adding the remaining extra-virgin olive oil, lemon zest and cayenne pepper to make a delicious lemony dressing. Drizzle the warm dressing over the perfectly cooked fish and veg and serve.

TIP
+ Za'atar (see page 242) works really well sprinkled on top of the cooked fish.

I love stuffing fish with delicious vegetables and herbs and serving them with a simple side of buttered greens and some lemon. Fish is a great source of Omega-3 fatty acids and although mullet isn't top of the list, it certainly has the full quota of amino acids which makes it a convenient source of protein. Leeks are a robust vegetable which suit roasting well, and also slightly caramelise, giving a lovely sweetness to complement the spicy rub on the fish. You don't need a barbecue and you won't be disappointed with the results.

Harissa Grilled Mullet

serves 2

---

1 whole red mullet (about 700g), gutted and descaled (you can ask your fishmonger or supermarket fish counter to do this for you)

4 tbsp extra-virgin olive oil

2 tsp harissa paste

8 thyme sprigs

leaves from 4 rosemary sprigs

1 lemon, cut into 3mm-thick slices

1 leek, washed, trimmed and roughly chopped

100g cherry tomatoes on the vine

100g asparagus spears

50g sugar snap peas

1 tsp butter

sea salt and freshly ground black pepper

Preheat the oven grill to medium.

Line a baking tray with foil and place the mullet on top. Score the flesh on both sides, making 1cm-deep cuts 4cm apart on both sides of the fish.

Rub the fish all over with 3 tablespoons of the oil and harissa, and season with salt and pepper. Stuff the cavity with the thyme, rosemary, lemon slices and leek and place the cherry tomatoes on the foil around the fish.

Grill the fish for 6–8 minutes on each side, waiting for the skin to brown before turning. The fish is cooked through if it flakes easily when gently prodded with a fork.

While the fish is under the grill, heat a pan over a medium heat. Snap any long asparagus in half so they fit into the pan and toss them in with the sugar snap peas. Season with salt and pepper, add the remaining tablespoon of olive oil and stir for 1–2 minutes. Splash in 20ml water and cover with a lid for 2 minutes. Uncover and make sure the water has evaporated. Serve them coated in butter.

TIPS

+ Try this stuffed, grilled fish recipe with other types of fish, such as mackerel, sea bass or red snapper.
+ You could cook the fish on a barbecue if you wish, by putting the fish in a fish 'cage' and grilling it on both sides, as above.

Mains

Trout is prized for its high Omega-3 content and pairs beautifully with Asian flavours. Wasabi and ginger make a beautiful dressing: their volatile compounds are known for their antioxidant capacity and ability to fight bacteria. It's thought to be the reason why the Japanese traditionally paired them with sushi, to prevent the raw fish from turning.

Sesame-crusted Trout with Wasabi and Ginger Dressing

serves 2

100g pak choy, thinly sliced

100g snow pea shoots, roughly sliced (or watercress, beansprouts or spinach)

100g red cabbage, finely shredded

300g boneless trout fillets

2 tbsp coconut oil, melted

drizzle of soy sauce

20g sesame seeds

100g edamame bean noodles or whole soba noodles

For the wasabi and ginger dressing

3cm piece of root ginger, peeled and grated

3cm piece of fresh wasabi (or horseradish), grated

3 tsp rice wine (or honey)

1 tbsp soy sauce

grated zest and juice of 1 lime

2 tbsp sesame oil (or melted coconut oil)

Preheat the oven to 200°C/180°C fan/gas 6.

Put the pak choy, snow pea shoots and red cabbage in a bowl and toss together.

Smother the trout fillets with the coconut oil, drizzle with the soy sauce and coat them on both sides with the sesame seeds.

Heat an ovenproof frying pan over a medium heat, and dry-fry the fish skin-side down for 2–3 minutes, until the skin crisps up. Turn the fillets over and transfer the pan to the oven for 4 minutes, until the fish is just cooked through. (Transfer the fish to a baking dish if your frying pan isn't ovenproof.)

Cook the noodles in a pan of boiling water for 5 minutes (or according to the packet instructions), drain (or remove them from the water with tongs) and toss them through the raw vegetables in the bowl.

Combine the ingredients for the wasabi and ginger dressing in a bowl and pour it over the noodles and vegetables. Stack the fish fillets on top, and serve.

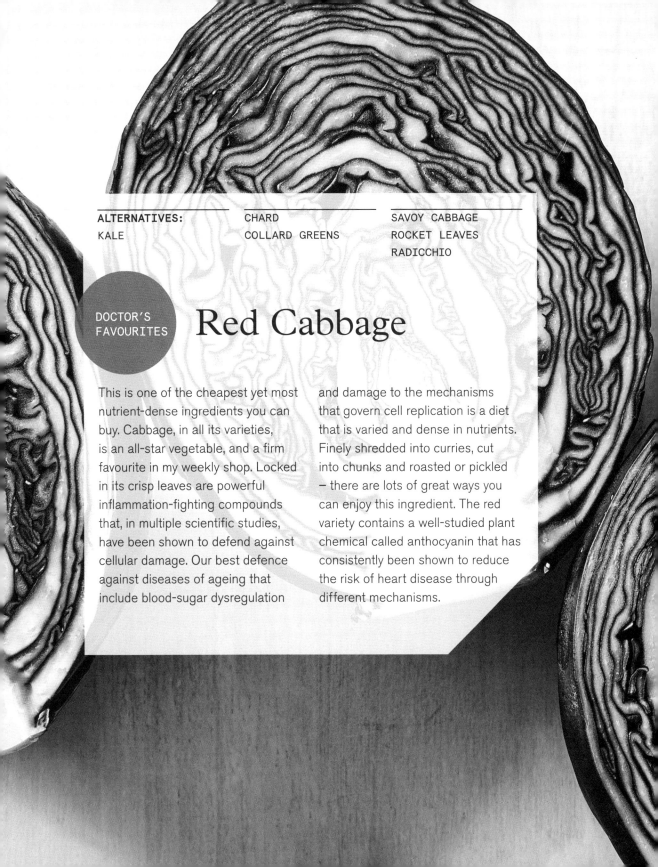

ALTERNATIVES:
KALE

CHARD
COLLARD GREENS

SAVOY CABBAGE
ROCKET LEAVES
RADICCHIO

DOCTOR'S
FAVOURITES

Red Cabbage

This is one of the cheapest yet most nutrient-dense ingredients you can buy. Cabbage, in all its varieties, is an all-star vegetable, and a firm favourite in my weekly shop. Locked in its crisp leaves are powerful inflammation-fighting compounds that, in multiple scientific studies, have been shown to defend against cellular damage. Our best defence against diseases of ageing that include blood-sugar dysregulation and damage to the mechanisms that govern cell replication is a diet that is varied and dense in nutrients. Finely shredded into curries, cut into chunks and roasted or pickled – there are lots of great ways you can enjoy this ingredient. The red variety contains a well-studied plant chemical called anthocyanin that has consistently been shown to reduce the risk of heart disease through different mechanisms.

The stars of this dish are the vibrant smoky vegetables and comforting bean purée, complemented by perfect pan-fried chicken cooked in herbs. I eat chicken about once a week, and quite often in a comforting dish such as this. I encourage consuming a moderate amount of fats like those found in chicken skin and butter, as they form part of a very healthy diet and add a wealth of flavour. Also, it's preferable to choose sources of protein and fat from whole foods than to spend money on collagen supplements, vitamins and other pills that don't have a clear evidence base for their use.

Sautéed Parsnips, Bean Purée and Pan-fried Chicken

serves 2
with leftovers

3 tbsp extra-virgin olive oil

150g parsnips, cut into 2cm cubes (unpeeled)

3 garlic cloves, roughly chopped

½ tsp cayenne pepper

1 tsp smoked sweet paprika

100g Brussels sprouts, roughly chopped

100g cavolo nero, roughly chopped

300g skin-on chicken breasts

20g butter

5g sage leaves, finely chopped

50g watercress, roughly chopped

sea salt and freshly ground black pepper

For the bean purée

400g tin cannellini beans, drained and rinsed

1 garlic clove

juice of ½ lemon

20ml hot water

To make the bean purée, put the beans, garlic, lemon juice and water in a blender or food processor, season with salt and pepper and blitz until smooth. Set aside.

Heat 2 tablespoons of oil in a frying pan or saucepan over a medium heat, add the parsnips and sauté for 4 minutes, then add the garlic, cayenne and paprika and cook for a further 4 minutes. Toss in the Brussels sprouts and cavolo nero and cook for 3 minutes, then cover and continue to cook for 2 minutes. Remove from the heat.

Heat a dry frying pan over a medium heat. Flatten the chicken breasts by placing them between two sheets of baking parchment and beating them with a rolling pin.

Season both sides of the chicken breasts, drizzle with the remaining oil and place them skin-side down in the pan. Gently press them in the pan to help the skin crisp up and cook for 5–6 minutes, then turn them over. Add the butter and sage to the pan and baste the breasts with the sage butter for 3–4 minutes, until cooked through (the meat should not be pink, and the juices should run clear).

Remove the chicken breasts from the pan and allow to rest for a few minutes, then slice them and serve them on top of the bean purée, with the watercress and sautéed parsnips alongside.

TIP
+ You can use skinless chicken breasts if you prefer.

Mains

Don't be put off by the long ingredients list – this recipe is deceptively simple to make and really satisfying. Beautifully marinated chicken is paired with a vibrant, crisp salad bursting with flavour and protective plant chemicals. If I had to choose my favourite salad leaf, it would have to be rocket. Part of the cruciferous family, it is a source of nitrates that are known to reduce inflammation in vessels, reduce blood pressure and protect against cancer. The bitter taste of the rocket and the watercress's peppery edge are balanced out by the sweet apple.

Rosemary and Fennel Chicken with Herby Lemon Dressing

serves 2

300g skinless, boneless
    chicken thighs

75g green beans

50g watercress, roughly chopped

50g rocket, finely chopped

50g apple, thinly sliced (unpeeled)

sea salt and freshly ground
    black pepper

For the marinade

3 tbsp extra-virgin olive oil

1 tsp finely chopped
    rosemary needles

1 tsp ground fennel seeds

grated zest and juice of 1 lemon

3 garlic cloves, grated

For the herby lemon dressing

10g mint leaves, finely chopped

10g flat-leaf parsley, leaves
    and stalks finely chopped

20ml extra-virgin olive oil

1 red chilli, deseeded and
    thinly sliced

grated zest and juice of 1 lemon

2 garlic cloves, grated

Combine the marinade ingredients in a bowl and season with salt and pepper, then add the chicken thighs, coat them in the mixture and leave to marinate for at least 20 minutes (ideally overnight, covered, in the fridge).

Heat a dry frying pan over a medium heat and place the marinated chicken thighs in the pan. Cook for 6 minutes, until the meat browns, gently pressing the thighs in the pan to encourage them to colour, then turn them over and cook for a further 2–3 minutes until cooked through (the meat should not be pink, and the juices should run clear). Transfer them to a plate and leave to rest, covered, while you prepare the rest of the dish.

Steam the green beans for 2 minutes with a pinch of salt (you can use the 'perfect' method on page 102), then put them in a large bowl (while they're still hot), add the watercress, rocket and apple and toss to combine.

Combine the dressing ingredients in a bowl and season with salt and pepper, then drizzle it over the salad.

Roughly slice the chicken and serve with the salad.

TIP
+ Serve with plain roasted sweet potato or butternut squash to make this a complete meal.

Mains

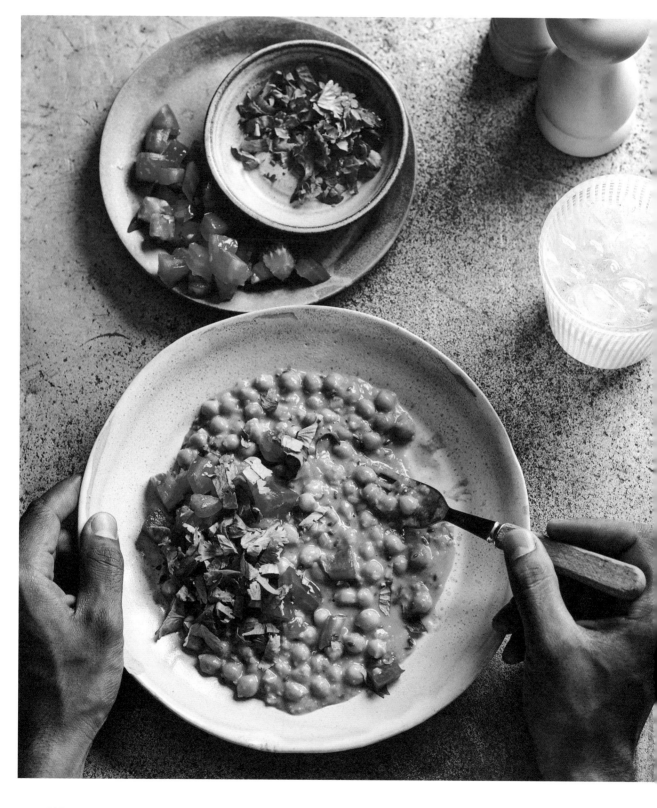

Mains

This fusion dish combines two cuisines that you might think are incompatible: South American and Indian. Humitas, a South American dish, is a delicious sweetcorn porridge made with lots of milk, butter and paprika and I've discovered that the flavour of sweetcorn goes really well with chickpeas and Indian spices. This dish will turn your perception of curry on its head! Chickpeas are one of my favourite plant-based sources of protein, with the added bonus of fibre, offering essential nutrients to keep your cells functioning efficiently and encourage a healthy population of gut microbes. I like to serve it with a small portion of wild rice and lots of spinach.

Sweetcorn Chana Curry

serves 2

1 sweetcorn cob (150g)

2 tbsp coconut oil

½ white onion, finely chopped

¼ tsp turmeric

1 tsp cumin seeds

1 tsp coriander seeds

1 star anise

½ tsp chilli powder

400g tin chickpeas, drained and rinsed (or 200g dried chickpeas, cooked 'perfectly' – see page 96)

50ml coconut cream

sea salt and freshly ground black pepper

1 large tomato, finely diced, to serve

small bunch of coriander, leaves and stalks finely chopped, to serve

Grate the sweetcorn cob into a bowl using a box grater. It should be liquid and creamy.

Melt the coconut oil in a saucepan over a medium heat, add the onion, turmeric, cumin and coriander seeds and star anise and sauté for a few minutes until the onion has softened. Stir in the chilli powder and grated sweetcorn and cook for 2 minutes, to infuse the corn with the flavour of the spices, then add the chickpeas and coconut cream and simmer for 6–8 minutes until soft and creamy. Season with salt and pepper to taste.

Serve the sweetcorn curry garnished with the diced tomato and chopped coriander.

TIPS

+ 2 teaspoons of my garam masala (see page 240) would also work well instead of using cumin, coriander seeds and star anise.
+ This goes really well with a portion of cooked wild rice (see page 100) and roughly chopped spinach.

I love making different pastes, marinades and chutneys. They're a fantastic and enjoyable way to introduce a variety of plant chemicals into your diet. The apple and pea chutney is a product of endless experimenting with ingredients in my family kitchen and it's bursting with protein and the antioxidants we find in the humble apple. Using Greek yoghurt in the marinade for this easy chicken dish gives the meat a lovely crust when cooked.

Spiced Chicken Skewers with Apple and Pea Chutney

serves 2

300g boneless, skinless chicken thighs, cut into 4cm cubes

1 tsp coconut oil

1 red onion, thinly sliced

5cm piece of root ginger, peeled and grated

2 green cardamom pods

100g spinach, finely chopped

25g cherry tomatoes, halved

15g coriander, leaves and stalks finely chopped

sea salt and black pepper

For the marinade

3 garlic cloves

4cm piece of root ginger, peeled

1 green chilli, deseeded

25g Greek yoghurt

1 tsp each ground cumin, ground fennel and ground cinnamon

For the apple and pea chutney

1 apple, cored and roughly chopped

15g coriander, leaves and stalks

grated zest and juice of 1 lime

1 red chilli, deseeded

75g peas (fresh or thawed)

To make the marinade, blend the garlic, ginger and chilli in a blender or food processor until finely chopped. Transfer to a bowl, add the yoghurt, cumin, fennel and cinnamon, season well and mix. Add the chicken pieces, and coat them in the marinade. Leave for at least 20 minutes (ideally overnight, covered, in the fridge).

Preheat the grill to medium.

Push the marinated chicken pieces onto the skewers and line them on a rack under the grill. Cook for 22–25 minutes, until lightly charred, turning them halfway through to ensure they cook evenly.

While the chicken skewers are cooking, melt the coconut oil in a saucepan over a medium heat, add the onion, ginger and cardamom pods and sauté for 1–2 minutes until soft. Fold in the spinach, tomatoes and coriander, cover with a lid then remove from the heat.

To make the chutney, blitz the apple, coriander, lime zest and juice, red chilli and peas in a blender or food processor until roughly blended. Add a splash of water to loosen if needed.

Serve the chicken skewers with the sautéed spinach and chutney.

TIP
+ Serve with perfectly cooked wholegrain or wild rice with a clove in the cooking water for flavour (see page 100).

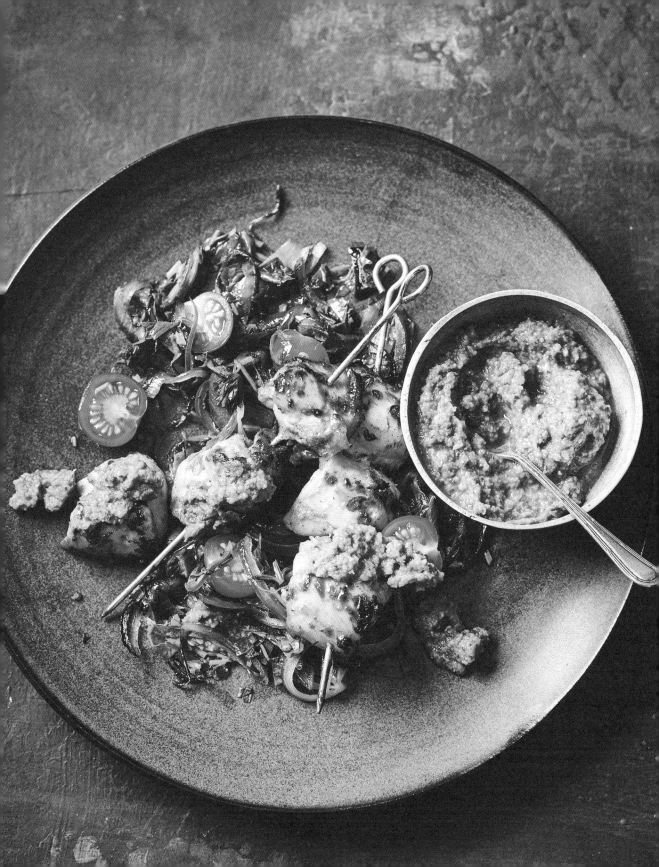

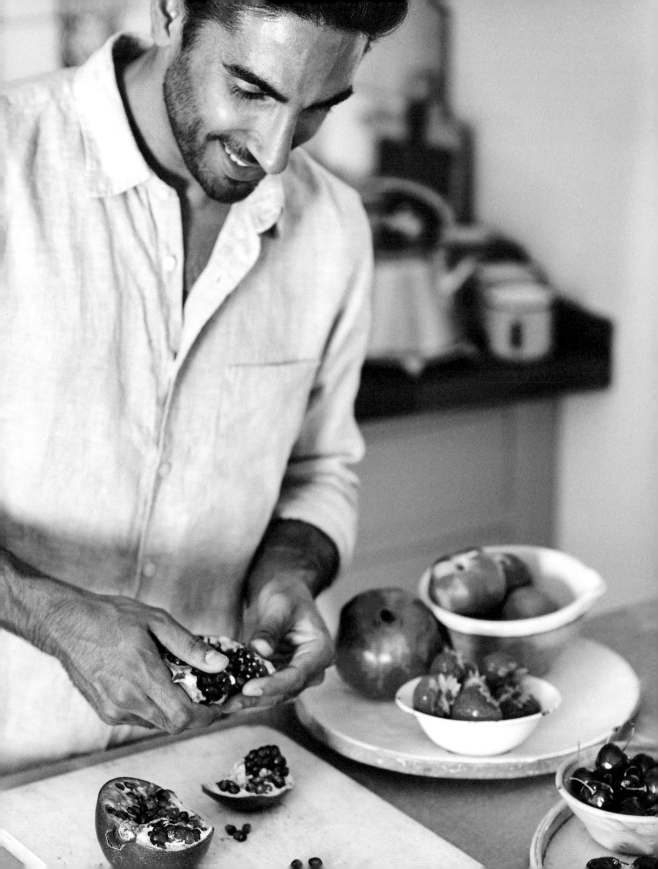

Desserts

Unless I manage to get home in time for dinner (which isn't often), I rarely muster enough energy to make a 'full-on' dessert, as well as a proper meal. My 'sweet' usually consists of a spoonful of good-quality nut butter with grated dark chocolate and some whole fruit. However, here are a few puddings, for when you have the time to indulge in something a little more luxurious.

'Healthy' pancakes usually don't fit the bill for me. Gluten-free flour and chalky protein powders are not ingredients that find themselves in my cupboard. Instead, when I have a craving for a satisfying, sweet dessert I like using wholesome ingredients. Hemp seeds are a 'health food' that I think is worth the extra cost, because of its high protein content and nutty texture and flavour. The seeds work so well with sweet banana and cinnamon in this American-style pancake recipe.

Cinnamon Hemp Pancakes

serves 2

1 egg, beaten

2 tbsp shelled hemp seeds (or ground flaxseed), plus extra to serve

2 bananas, 1 mashed, 1 sliced

1 tsp ground cinnamon

1 tbsp coconut flour (or almond flour/another nut flour)

1 tbsp plain flour (or buckwheat, if gluten free)

30–40ml almond milk (or dairy/coconut milk)

1 tsp baking powder

2 tbsp coconut oil

1 tbsp maple syrup

15g shelled, unsalted pistachios, toasted and lightly crushed

Combine the egg, hemp seeds, mashed banana, cinnamon, both flours, milk and baking powder in a bowl. For American-style pancakes, you want to achieve a 'dropping' consistency; add a further 20–30ml milk if you like thinner pancakes.

Melt the coconut oil in a large frying pan over a medium heat, then pour 2 tablespoons of batter into the pan (pour another 2 tablespoons of batter into the pan if it will accommodate it — you should have enough batter for 4 pancakes). Fry the pancakes, in batches if necessary, for 1–2 minutes on each side, until lightly browned.

Stack the warm pancakes on a plate and drizzle with the maple syrup, scatter over the crushed pistachios and some extra hemp seeds, and top with the sliced banana.

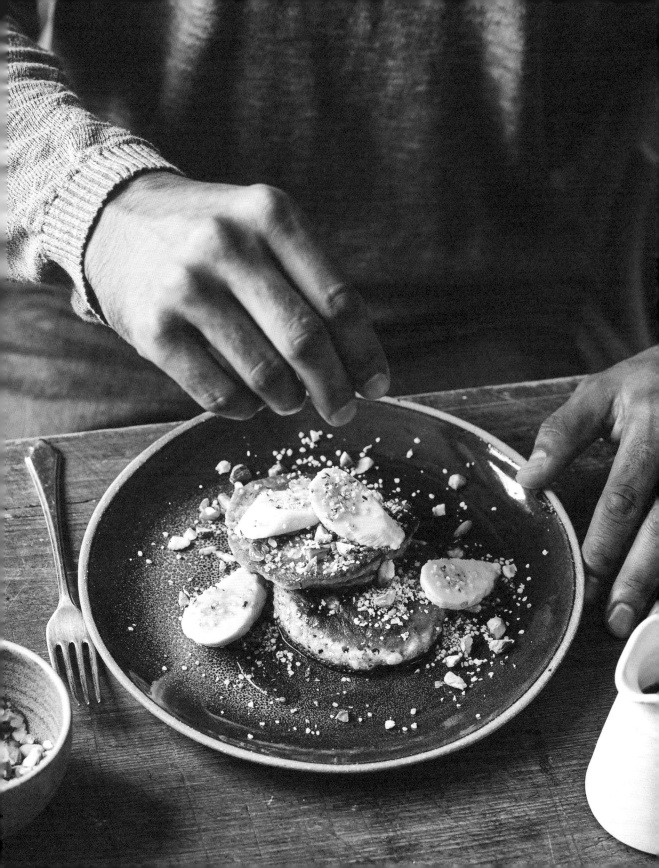

Matcha green tea has a distinctive aroma and taste. Just like red wine and dark chocolate, the complex flavour is due to the immense concentration of plant chemicals like catechins. These are what give matcha its potential health benefits and it's worth acquiring a taste for. But don't forget about the phytonutrient density of the humble apple. Lightly cooking it releases some of those plant chemicals known to be beneficial for our health. The apple's sweetness also mellows matcha's bitterness, and wholesome rice with almond milk is a comforting mixture that pairs well with all these flavours.

Apple and Matcha
Rice Pudding

serves 2

200g wholegrain rice (red or black), cooked 'perfectly' (see pages 99–100)

200ml almond milk (or milk of choice)

2 tsp honey, plus extra to serve

2 apples, cored and finely diced (unpeeled)

2 tsp matcha green tea powder, plus extra to serve

Put the rice in a pan with the almond milk, honey and half the diced apple and simmer for 5 minutes.

Remove from the heat and stir in the matcha powder. Allow to cool a little and then pour into bowls, scatter the remaining diced apple on top and dust with extra matcha and a drizzle of honey.

TIPS

+ Stir roughly 1 tablespoon of shelled hemp seeds into the pan when you add the matcha powder to the rice and milk, for added protein.

+ Not a fan of matcha? Try 2 teaspoons of ground cinnamon instead with some chopped dates, or perhaps cacao powder and some chopped banana.

Desserts

I'm not going to attempt to recreate my mother's kheer recipe. It's like an Indian rice pudding and is made with full-fat milk, coconut and tons of sugar. It's delightful! Instead, I make a similar version with just as much exotic spice, and using white quinoa and almond milk. Trust me, quinoa tastes delicious in a sweet recipe, but the spices are key. Cinnamon, nutmeg and cardamom are gorgeous, antioxidant-rich spices that are the perfect mix for Indian rice pudding. A couple of dried fruits and honey offer an earthy sweetness. Serve this with fruits such as mango slices or fresh berries.

serves 2
generously

Quinoa Kheer

100g cooked white quinoa (see page 100)

3 saffron strands (optional)

250ml almond milk (or other milk of choice)

1 tbsp runny honey

10g raisins or sultanas

½ tsp ground cinnamon, plus extra to serve

3 green cardamom pods, lightly crushed

pinch of ground or freshly grated nutmeg

1 tbsp ground flaxseed

10g shelled, unsalted pistachios, toasted and finely crushed

2 tsp desiccated coconut

Combine the quinoa, saffron (if using) and almond milk in a saucepan with the honey, raisins, cinnamon, cardamom pods, nutmeg and flaxseeds. Bring to a simmer over a low heat for 4–5 minutes, stirring until thickened, then remove from the heat.

Scatter with the crushed pistachios, a dusting of cinnamon and the desiccated coconut to serve.

TIPS

+ Swap the saffron for dried rose petals, to add a delicate perfume to the dish.
+ Use 1 tablespoon chia seeds instead of flaxseeds to give the dish a more gelatinous quality.
+ You can use any dried fruit you prefer, such as prunes or dates.

Desserts

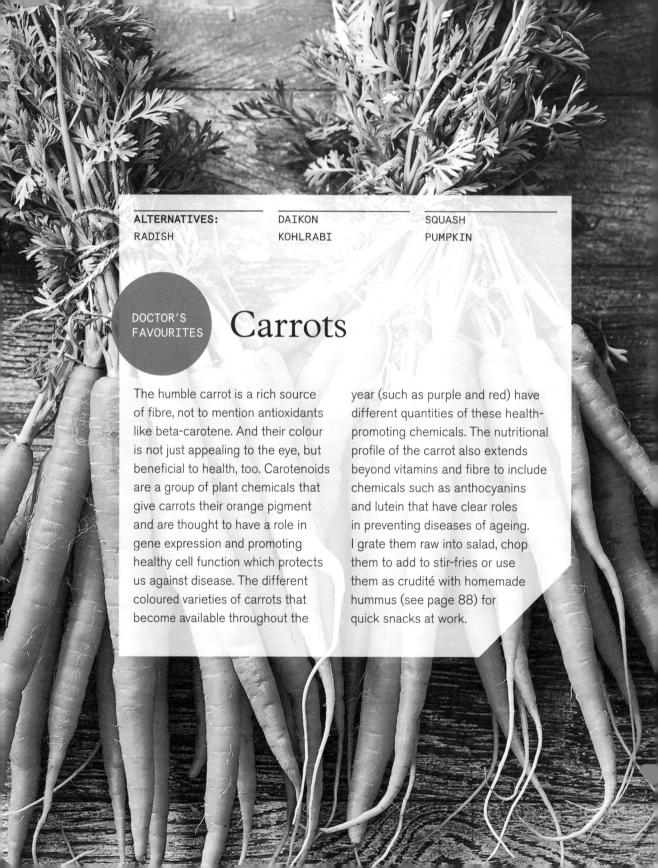

DOCTOR'S
FAVOURITES

Carrots

The humble carrot is a rich source of fibre, not to mention antioxidants like beta-carotene. And their colour is not just appealing to the eye, but beneficial to health, too. Carotenoids are a group of plant chemicals that give carrots their orange pigment and are thought to have a role in gene expression and promoting healthy cell function which protects us against disease. The different coloured varieties of carrots that become available throughout the year (such as purple and red) have different quantities of these health-promoting chemicals. The nutritional profile of the carrot also extends beyond vitamins and fibre to include chemicals such as anthocyanins and lutein that have clear roles in preventing diseases of ageing. I grate them raw into salad, chop them to add to stir-fries or use them as crudité with homemade hummus (see page 88) for quick snacks at work.

One of the most magical sights on a trip to India (or even your local high-street Asian confectioner) is a sweetshop counter, laden with all the colours, smells and sickly-sweet tastes you could imagine. They are probably the unhealthiest element of the Asian diet and our indulgence is in part responsible for a lot of diabetic cases. But at the heart of Indian desserts are wholesome healthy ingredients – I believe we need to retrain our taste buds to appreciate the complex beauty of spice, which has been blunted by adding lashings of sugar. This elegant, flavourful dessert showcases how nutrient-dense 'everyday' foods can be transformed into incredible treats. Carrot's natural sugars caramelise and are perfectly complemented by the tarry texture of dates. A rich source of beta-carotene, they also contain fibre, and pistachios are full of potassium and phytosterols that may have positive effects on blood pressure.

Coconut Gajar Halwa

serves 2

2 tbsp coconut oil

1 cinnamon stick (or a few pieces of cinnamon bark), broken in two

3 green cardamom pods, crushed

30g shelled, unsalted pistachios, toasted and lightly crushed

2 carrots (about 150g), grated

1 apple (about 100g), cored and grated (unpeeled)

2–3 dates, finely chopped (or dried raisins or sultanas)

25g coconut cream

150ml almond milk (or milk of choice, or water)

1 tsp ground cinnamon

2 tbsp hemp seeds

exotic fresh fruit, to serve

Melt the coconut oil in a frying pan over a medium heat, add the broken cinnamon stick, crushed cardamom pods and pistachios and toast them in the oil for 1–2 minutes.

Add the grated carrot, apple and dates to the pan and sauté for 2 minutes until softened, then add the coconut cream and almond milk, stir and simmer very gently for 3 minutes.

Remove from the heat and transfer to serving bowls, then dust with the cinnamon and scatter with the hemp seeds. Serve with fresh, exotic fruit.

This smooth, creamy delight is easy to whip up and made of unusual but incredibly healthy ingredients that taste amazing. Tofu is a great calcium source which is vital for your cells to function. Pomegranate gives the dessert a floral flavour with a sharp, tangy bite, and pistachios are a delicious heart-healthy nut. This is a great crowd pleaser for dinner parties and easy to prepare in advance.

Coconut Ice with Pomegranate and Caramel Pistachios

serves 2–3

300g smooth silken tofu

150g coconut cream

2 ripe bananas, peeled

handful of pomegranate seeds

20g shelled, unsalted pistachios, lightly crushed

1 tbsp honey

Put the tofu, coconut cream and bananas in a blender or food processor and blitz until smooth. Transfer to a large bowl and fold through the pomegranate seeds. Cover and transfer to the freezer for 2–3 hours: 2 hours will give you ice cream with a frozen-yoghurt-style soft-set texture, and 3 hours will give it a harder set.

Before serving, toast the crushed pistachios in a dry frying pan over a medium heat until brown, then remove from the heat and drizzle honey over them to slightly caramelise them. Leave to cool and become crumbly.

Top the tofu ice cream with the caramelised pistachios.

TIPS
+ Chopped red grapes can be used instead of pomegranate seeds.
+ Try experimenting with what's in season, such as blackberries and raspberries.

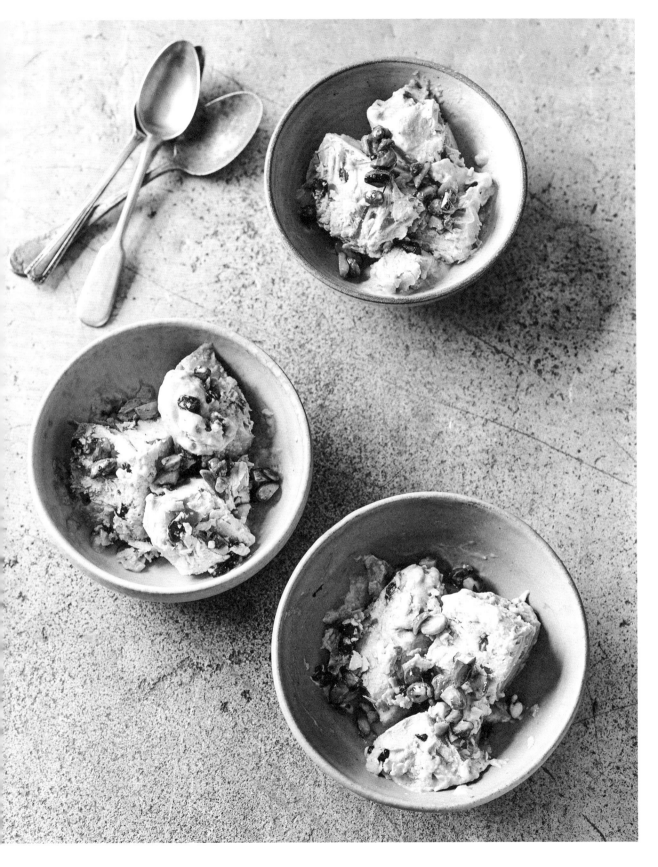

I have no problem using good-quality dairy products but this plant-based recipe is absolutely delightful. The sweet banana brings the matcha to life and the hint of ginger works very well with citrus. It's another easy way of getting one of my favourite medicinal spices – ginger – into the diet. This bowl of goodness is really well balanced.

Matcha and Ginger Ice Cream

serves 2–3

3 ripe bananas, peeled and chopped

300g smooth silken tofu

2 tsp matcha green tea powder

1 tsp grated root ginger

grated zest and juice of 1 lime

1 tsp honey

10g walnuts, toasted and lightly crushed

Put all the ingredients (except the walnuts) in a blender or food processor and blitz until smooth.

Pour into a flat tray and transfer to the freezer for 2 hours until softly set. Don't overfreeze it, as it will lose the silky texture.

Serve with the crushed walnuts scattered on top.

TIPS

+ Try 1 teaspoon ground cinnamon and 2 teaspoons cacao powder in place of the matcha.
+ Experiment with different nuts, such as peanuts or pistachios.

Here's another simple way to consume the incredible polyphenols in ginger and lime. This is one of my favourite tricks that I always keep in the freezer ready to jazz up simple fruits. I use saffron purely as a colouring agent here, rather than for its potential effect on reducing inflammation. For now, these delicate strands simply turn this dessert into a feast for the eyes.

Ginger and Cardamom Granita

serves 2

thumb-sized piece of root ginger, peeled and finely grated

seeds from 3 green cardamom pods, lightly ground

grated zest and juice of 1 lime

300ml water

2 tbsp honey

2–3 saffron strands

fresh fruit and berries, to serve

a few mint leaves, to serve

Put all the ingredients (except the fresh fruit and mint) in a saucepan and bring to the boil. Simmer for a few minutes then pour the mixture into a flat tray that will fit in the freezer.

Cover with baking parchment and when cooled, transfer to the freezer for 2–3 hours. Scrape the granita with a fork to break up the ice crystals and serve it with fruits and berries. Garnish with fresh mint.

TIPS

+ Use the tiniest pinch of ground turmeric to colour the granita if you don't have saffron.
+ Use 1 teaspoon of ground cardamom if you can't find fresh pods.

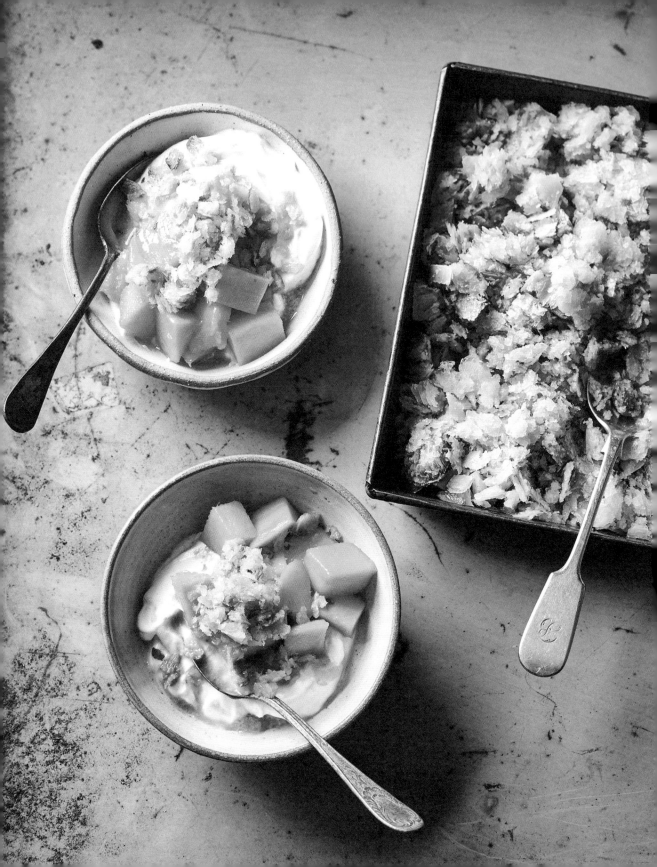

Vitamin C in citrus fruit boosts the availability of phytonutrient compounds in matcha, making this a refreshing and inflammation-fighting dessert. The slightly bitter flavour of matcha is sensational when paired with sweet, exotic fruit such as pineapple or mango and probiotic yoghurt. I also serve it as a palate cleanser and to top tequila-based cocktails!

Matcha and Lemongrass Granita

serves 2

150ml water

150ml almond milk (or cashew/
   oat milk)

1 tsp matcha green tea powder

2 tbsp honey

grated zest and juice of ½ lime

3cm piece of lemongrass (tender
   base only), bruised

probiotic yoghurt and sliced exotic
   fruit, to serve

Warm the water and almond milk in a saucepan over a medium heat, then stir in the matcha tea, honey, lime juice and zest and lemongrass. Once hot (but not boiling), pour the mixture into a flat tray that will fit in the freezer.

Cover with baking parchment and when cooled, remove the lemongrass and transfer to the freezer for 2–3 hours.

Scrape the granita with a fork to break up the ice crystals and spoon it on top of probiotic yogurt and sliced exotic fruit.

TIPS

+ Use the grated zest and juice of 1 whole lime (instead of just the ½ lime) if you can't get hold of fresh lemongrass.
+ This granita tastes just as delicious with apple or orange, if exotic fruit is unavailable.
+ Try using a different tea: rose and Earl Grey or jasmine tea work well. Add an extra spoon of honey to counter the bitterness if needed.

Ever since I came across a paper examining the increased antioxidant effect of adzuki beans coupled with raspberries, I always thought it would be fun to create a recipe that featured both of them. Adzuki bean is a delicious ingredient commonly found in Japanese desserts and savoury dishes. It's very high in both protein and fibre (similar to black beans). I've paired the rich flavour of adzuki with raspberries, prunes and cacao to create an indulgent dessert that should be treated as such: sugar from prunes, or raw cane sugar, is just as harmful in excess as the refined white stuff. These slices are 'healthier' than most, due to their protein, fibre and antioxidants, but try not to gorge!

Raspberry Adzuki Slices

serves 6

coconut oil, for greasing

250g fresh or frozen raspberries

250g pitted prunes

400g tin adzuki beans, drained and rinsed (or 150g dried adzuki beans, cooked 'perfectly' – see page 97)

2 tbsp cacao powder

3 tbsp coconut flour, almond flour or other nut flour

½ tsp baking powder

coconut yoghurt or ice cream, to serve

Preheat the oven to 200°C/180°C fan/gas 6, line a 20cm x 20cm brownie tin with baking parchment and grease it with coconut oil.

Put all the ingredients in a blender or food processor and blitz until smooth. Transfer the mixture to the lined tin and bake in the oven for 30–35 minutes, until brown.

Remove from the oven and leave to cool in the tin, then remove and slice into small bites. Serve with coconut yoghurt or your favourite ice cream.

TIPS

+ If you can't find adzuki beans, black beans work just as well.
+ You can also use dates instead of prunes.

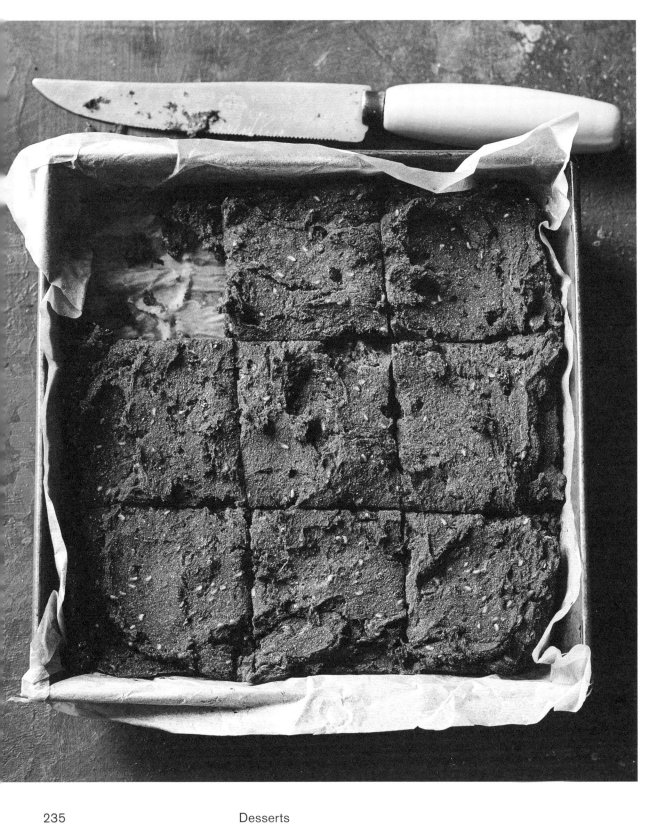

Desserts

The spices used in this easy yet indulgent dish are described in Ayurvedic practice as 'heat giving' and they certainly warm you up! I love eating this dessert on a cold winter evening or when I feel a cold coming on. I'll often make a teapot of these spices with some honey to settle my chest. Black peppercorns and ginger give the dish a subtle heat that marries well with clove and cardamom. It works perfectly with plain ice cream dusted with the apple skin 'crunch'.

Sweet Chai-spiced Apple with Pistachio Crunch

serves 2

2 apples, peel removed in long, thin strips

2 tsp coconut oil

2 tsp ground cinnamon

2 tsp demerara sugar

20g unsalted, shelled pistachios, toasted and finely crushed

400ml water

large piece of cinnamon bark or cinnamon stick

3 cloves

4 thin slices of root ginger (skin on)

4 black peppercorns (or ½ tsp ground black pepper)

generous pinch of freshly grated or ground nutmeg

4 green cardamom pods, lightly crushed

3 tbsp honey

Preheat the oven to 200°C/180°C fan/gas 6.

Rub the apple peel with the coconut oil, cinnamon and demerara sugar, place in a small roasting tin and bake for 8 minutes, or until lightly browned. Remove from the oven and allow to cool. The peel may still be slightly moist despite being nicely coloured, but it will firm up when cool and become crunchy. Roughly chop the peel, mix it with the crushed pistachios and set aside.

Pour the water into a saucepan with the cinnamon, cloves, ginger, peppercorns, nutmeg, cardamom and honey. Bring to a simmer and add the whole apples. Cover the pan with baking parchment and close the lid tightly over it, so no steam escapes. Cook over a low heat for 20 minutes, then remove from the heat. Transfer the apples to a bowl with a slotted spoon and continue to reduce the liquid until you have about 100ml left.

Serve the warm cooked apples drizzled with the chai syrup (I like to leave the aromatic whole spices in) and top with the apple 'crunch' and crushed pistachios.

TIP
+ This tastes great with frozen yoghurt or simple vanilla ice cream.

Desserts

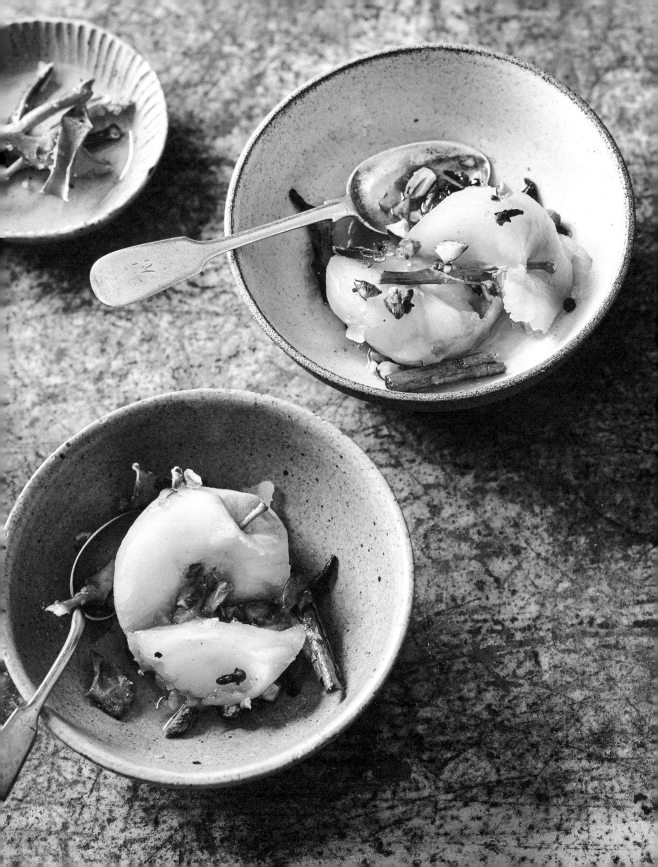

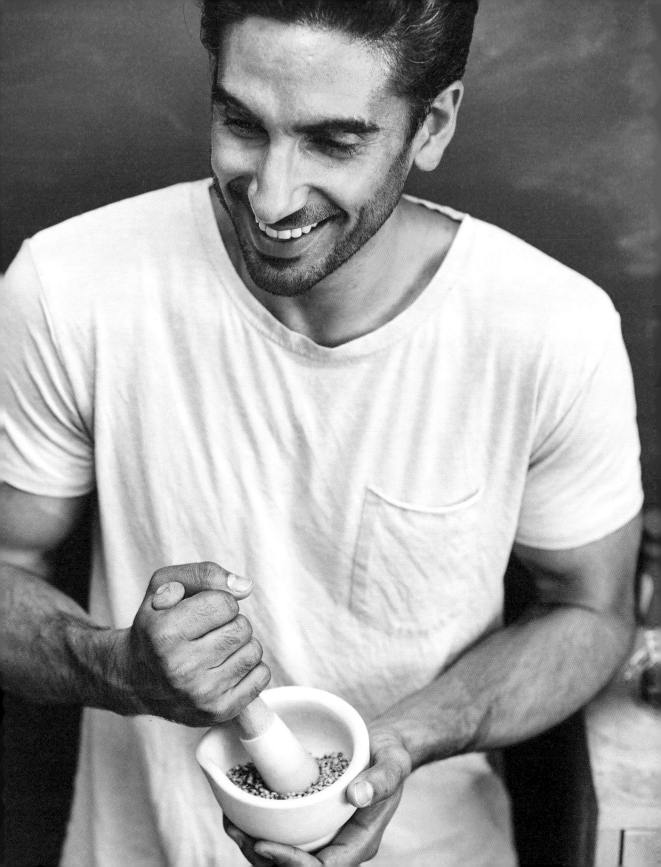

Spices, dressings and pastes

Some people bake, others like pickling and fermenting. I blend spices and make pastes: I like nothing better than creating a new barbecue rub with toasted seeds or experimenting with different oils for dressings. These simple touches elevate the most basic of ingredients. You can match any number of greens or legumes to my spice blends to create wonderful taste sensations. Keeping a paste in the fridge means you can transform a simple stir-fry into something special with minimal ingredients, and it finally gives you a use for all those empty nut-butter jars.

Every Indian family has a closely guarded secret recipe for their own garam masala blend. This is mine and I'm happy to share it. The spice mix is an antioxidant flavour bomb and I truly hope you mess around with different variations of it to make your own unique version. I choose to go heavier with the cloves than some do, as it's a spice with one of the highest antioxidant measures; it may be protective against cancer and it transforms this spice blend. It's easier to build heat into recipes as needed, rather than put dried chilli into the mix itself, so I choose to leave it out.

My Family's Secret Garam Masala

makes about 70g

2 tsp cloves

2 tsp cumin seeds

2 tsp fennel seeds

2 tsp freshly ground cinnamon bark (or ground cinnamon)

2 tsp seeds from black or green cardamom pods

2 tsp black peppercorns

4 star anise

6 dried or fresh bay leaves

Put all the ingredients in a dry frying pan and toast over a medium heat for 1–2 minutes until they start to release their aromas.

Transfer to a bowl and allow to cool, then tip into a coffee-bean grinder or pestle and mortar and grind to a coarse powder. Pass through a tea strainer if you want a finer spice powder.

Store the garam masala in an airtight container in a cool, dark place and use it within 3–4 weeks.

TIP

+ Melt 1 tablespoon of butter or ghee in a pan. Add 1 teaspoon of the garam masala, let it sizzle for a few seconds, then pour it into a vegetable stock to add an instant aromatic flavour. It works beautifully.

Spices, dressings and pastes

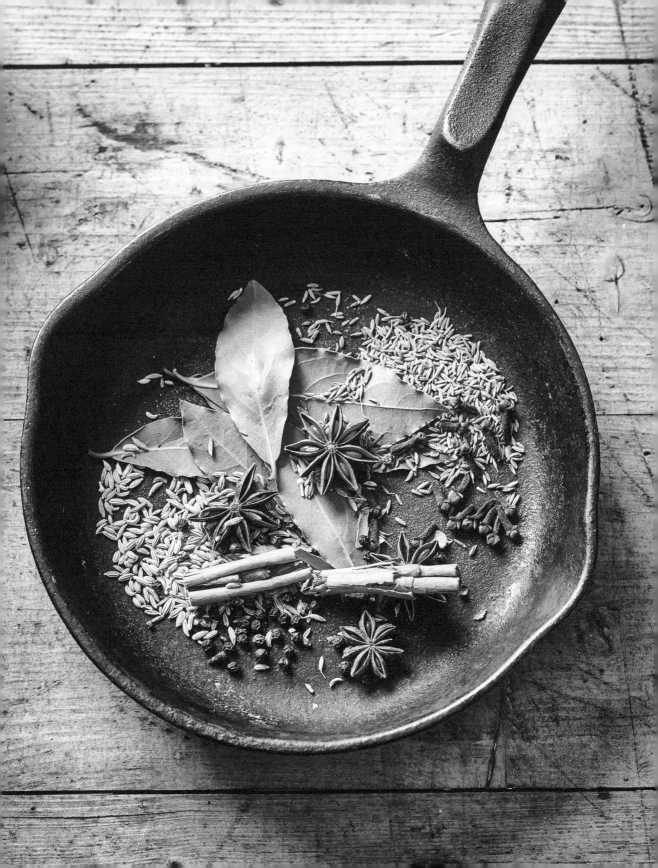

My good friend, who used to live in UAE, took me for a 'Lebanese pizza' when we arrived in Dubai during our medical elective. Essentially it was freshly made flatbread, a ton of olive oil and spoonfuls of beautiful herby za'atar. The moment I bit into the warm dough and experienced the sour tang of sumac with the hum of familiar thyme was unforgettable. Za'atar, an unparalleled mix of flavours, combines familiar kitchen herbs with exotic spices to create an entirely new taste sensation. It's the perfect way to use up fresh thyme that never made it from the fridge into a dish.

Za'atar Spice Blend

makes about 90g

4 tsp cumin seeds

4 tsp sesame seeds

4 tsp fresh or dried thyme leaves

4 tsp fresh or dried oregano leaves

6 tsp sumac

Put the cumin and sesame seeds in a dry frying pan and toast lightly over a medium heat for 1–2 minutes until they release their aromas.

Transfer to a bowl and allow to cool, then tip into a coffee-bean grinder or pestle and mortar and grind to a coarse powder.

Combine the ground spices with the rest of the ingredients and store the spice blend in an airtight container in a cool, dark place for up to 3–4 weeks.

TIPS

+ Mix 2 teaspoons of spice mixture with 30ml of extra-virgin olive oil for a brilliant herby salad dressing or even to flavour simple roast sweet potatoes.
+ You can gently dry fresh herbs in the oven on a low heat or buy them dry.

I'm lucky to have eaten my way all over America, including North Carolina, Florida, New Orleans and Chicago. I totally get America's love affair with barbecues. It's just so good! Sweet glazes combined with fresh herbs and spice hit so many taste receptors, but when you strip back the excessive sugar and the unnecessary use of salt, you're left with some pretty incredible ingredients. It's the indulgence in the sugar and salt that leads to the downfall of barbecue, so let's go back to basics and concentrate on flavour. Cumin, oregano and fennel are beautiful medicinal spices that aid digestion, and coriander seeds may even have positive effects on cholesterol ratios.

Best BBQ Blend

makes about 50g

2 tsp fennel seeds

2 tsp cumin seeds

2 tsp coriander seeds

2 tsp black peppercorns

2 tsp cayenne pepper

2 tsp smoked sweet paprika

2 tsp dried oregano

Put the fennel, cumin and coriander seeds and peppercorns in a dry frying pan and toast lightly over a medium heat for 1–2 minutes until they release their aromas.

Transfer to a bowl and allow to cool, then tip into a coffee-bean grinder or pestle and mortar and grind to a coarse powder.

Combine the ground spices with the rest of the ingredients and store in an airtight container in a cool, dark place for up to 3–4 weeks.

TIP

+ You can blend this spice mixture with extra-virgin olive oil before rubbing it into meat or even use it as a marinade. I sometimes use it as a dry rub with a little added salt and sugar for barbecues.

Spices, dressings and pastes

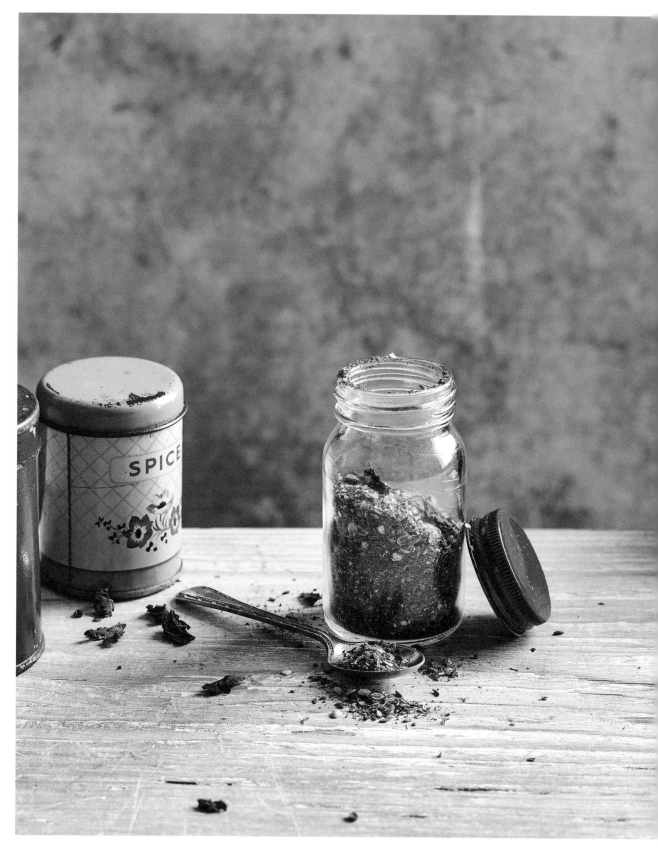

This North African spice blend carries amazing heat and an array of ingredients that pack a punch in both flavour and health benefits. It includes ingredients such as coriander and caraway seeds which are recognised for their antioxidant properties that protect us against degenerative disease. Pairing these blends with colourful vegetables of different varieties helps lower inflammation in the body which is linked to many conditions of ageing. I add rose petals to give it a delicate floral sweetness, but you can use palm sugar or coconut sugar instead, if you wish.

Rose Harissa

makes about 50g

2 tsp cumin seeds

2 tsp coriander seeds

2 tsp ground dried ancho chilli (or arbol, chipotle or plain dried chilli flakes)

1 tsp black peppercorns

2 tsp caraway seeds

2 tsp dried rose petals

2 tsp sweet paprika

Put the cumin and coriander seeds, chilli, peppercorns and caraway seeds in a dry frying pan and toast over a medium heat for 1–2 minutes until they release their aromas.

Transfer to a bowl and allow to cool, then tip into a coffee-bean grinder or pestle and mortar and grind to a coarse powder. Mix in the rose petals and paprika and store in an airtight container in a cool, dark place for up to 3–4 weeks.

TIPS

+ Blend 3 teaspoons with 50ml of extra-virgin olive oil to create a marinade for fish or chicken that you can simply bake or grill.
+ To make the spice mix into a paste, add a couple of tablespoons of water and a garlic clove and blend in a food processor.

Spices, dressings and pastes

Most people think pesto is unhealthy because of its fat content, but trust me, you want these types of fats in your diet. Whole nuts and seeds have been shown to have a positive effect on heart health, as has delicious extra-virgin olive oil. Basil is a herb rich in polyphenols that give it its distinctive bitter taste. This classic recipe will bring any soup to life, or try pairing it simply with green vegetables to help absorption of their fat-soluble vitamins.

Classic Pesto

makes about 50g

25g basil leaves

20g pine nuts

3 tbsp extra-virgin olive oil

sea salt and freshly ground
    black pepper

1–2 tsp grated Parmesan (optional)

Bruise the basil leaves in a pestle and mortar, then add the pine nuts and crush them before gradually pouring in the olive oil, mixing continuously. Stir in the salt, pepper and Parmesan (if using).

Alternatively, simply blitz the ingredients in a blender or food processor until they reach a rustic, yet velvety texture.

TIPS
+ Taste as you go along, to create the pesto you desire.
+ Get creative and swap the basil and pine nuts for different nuts, seeds and polyphenol-rich herbs, such as parsley or coriander, and macadamia nuts or pumpkin seeds.

Spices, dressings and pastes

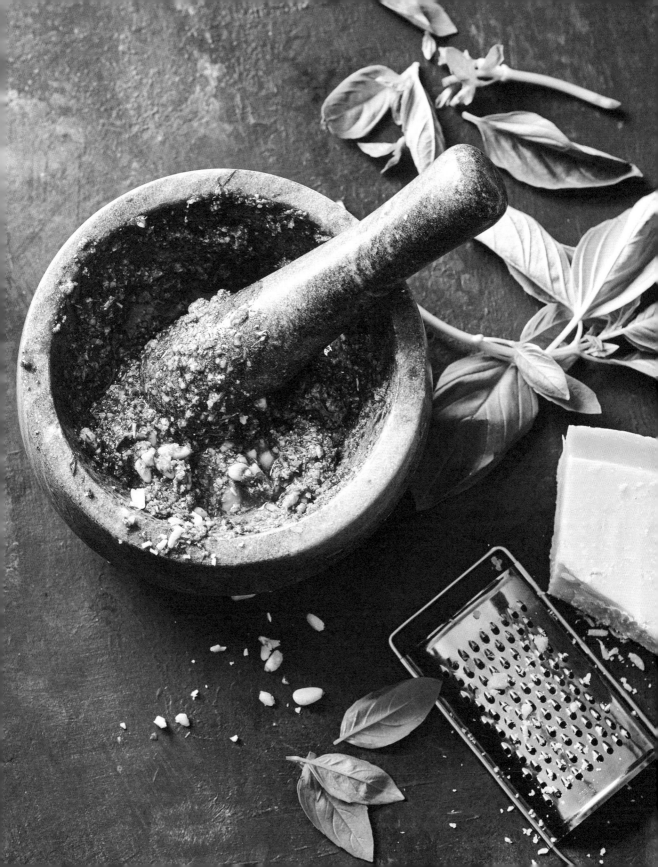

Set aside just half an hour to make this paste – it's really worth the effort. The explosion of freshness and flavour cannot be replicated by anything shop-bought. It has a similar aromatic element to garam masala (see page 240), but the addition of lemongrass and galangal makes it stand alone. Each ingredient offers a bundle of medicinal benefits supported by a growing body of research. Lemongrass fights cancer cells, garlic is what your gut bugs crave and cinnamon may reduce the release of chemicals related to ageing. All in all, this is full of fragrant, punchy, health-promoting compunds. In Vietnam I saw the garlic and galangal charred over charcoal, which adds a delicious, smoky aroma, but it's perhaps not the best way to release the precious volatile chemicals! Instead, I lightly toast them in a dry pan to release their oils.

Massaman Paste

makes about 30g

Dry spices

1 tsp fennel seeds

1 tsp cumin seeds

1 star anise

1 tsp black peppercorns

1 tsp seeds from green
   cardamom pods

1 tsp dried chilli flakes

1½ tsp ground cinnamon bark

Wet spices

4cm piece of lemongrass (tender
   base only), finely chopped

4 garlic cloves, roughly chopped

10g piece of galangal or ginger,
   peeled and finely chopped

2 shallots, finely chopped

Put the dry spices in a dry frying pan and toast lightly over a medium heat for 1–2 minutes until they release their aromas.

Transfer to a bowl and allow to cool, then tip into a coffee-bean grinder or pestle and mortar and grind to a fine powder. Tip them back into the bowl.

Put the wet spices in a dry frying pan and toast for 2–3 minutes, until they release their aromas and are lightly coloured, then transfer them to the pestle and mortar and pound for 10–15 minutes to form a paste, gradually adding the dry spices as you go. Alternatively, blend the toasted wet spices with the dry spices in a blender or food processor for a couple of minutes.

In my experience, using a pestle and mortar makes a much finer and more satisfying paste, but it requires a bit of elbow grease!

Store the paste in an airtight container in the fridge for up to 4 weeks.

TIP

+ All Massaman pastes need coconut cream and a bit of sweetness added at the time of cooking. Try this paste in my Butternut Massaman Curry on page 203.

You don't need to travel to the Caribbean to experience the beauty of authentic Jerk. One of my earliest memories of Caribbean cuisine was the first time I tried Jerk chicken, at Notting Hill Carnival. I thought growing up eating spicy Indian food would give me a decent level of immunity to the heat of Scotch bonnet and habanero chilli. I was wrong. On sinking my teeth into the charred chicken, the searing heat hit my senses immediately! This recipe is lighter on the chilli, but heavier on the beautiful aromatic components that give Jerk its wonderful complexity.

makes about 60g # Jerk Paste

½ red onion, roughly chopped

1 garlic clove, roughly chopped

thumb-sized piece of root ginger, peeled and roughly chopped

1 habanero chilli (or 1 red chilli), deseeded

1 tsp ground cinnamon

1 tsp ground allspice

¼ tsp freshly grated nutmeg

1 tsp freshly ground black pepper

1 tsp dark brown sugar

leaves from 8 thyme sprigs

Put the onion, garlic, ginger and chilli in a dry frying pan and toast over a medium heat for 3–4 minutes, to release their aromas, then transfer them to a pestle and mortar or a blender with the remaining ingredients and pound or blitz to form a paste.

Store the paste in an airtight container in the fridge for up to 3–4 weeks.

TIP

+ To make a Jerk-style sauce, mix 2 teaspoons of the paste with 100g tinned chopped tomatoes, the juice of 1 lime, 3 teaspoons of red wine vinegar and 1 teaspoon of tomato purée in a pan, and simmer for 15 minutes until thick and reduced.

Spices, dressings and pastes

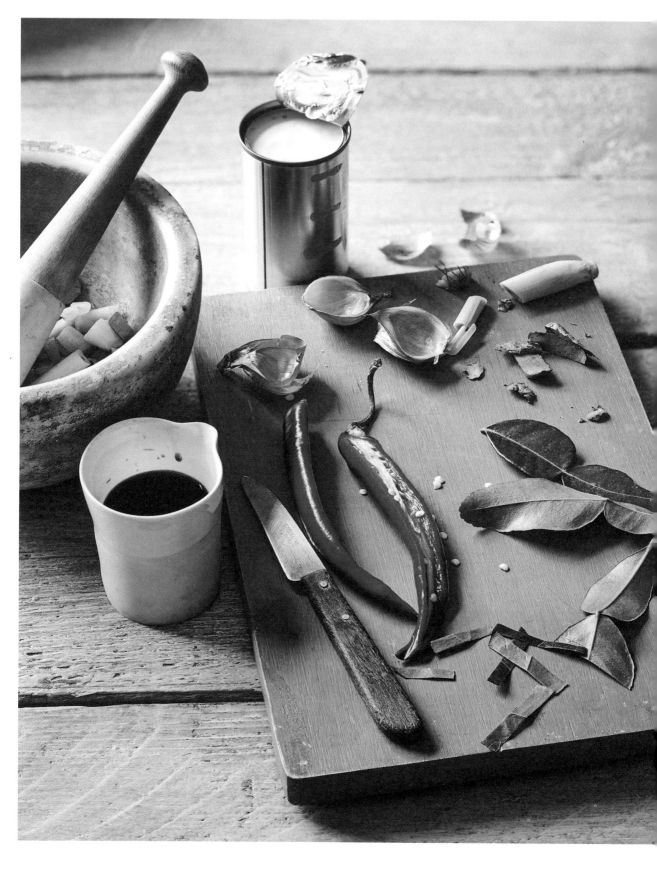

Lemongrass is a fragrant and hugely potent spice which packs a big antioxidant punch. I use it in Southeast Asian cooking and Indian curries, but don't shy away from using it in other dishes too. It adds a citrus note to rice, noodles or even plain lentils. To help me wind down after a busy shift, I sometimes put a bruised stick into a mug of plain hot water and use it as a stirrer, letting its oils gently release into my drink. You can add this paste to coconut or almond milk to make a luxuriously rich sauce to poach fish in or add to steamed vegetables.

Lemongrass and Turmeric Paste

makes about 50g

6cm piece of lemongrass (tender base only), roughly chopped

1 shallot, roughly chopped

4cm piece of turmeric root, peeled and chopped (or 2 tsp ground turmeric)

3 garlic cloves, roughly chopped

1 red chilli, deseeded and chopped

2 dried or fresh kaffir lime leaves, roughly chopped

1 tbsp soy sauce

4 drops of fish sauce (optional)

2 tbsp coconut cream

Put the lemongrass, shallot, turmeric (if using fresh) and garlic in a dry frying pan and toast over a medium heat for 2–3 minutes, to release their aromas.

Transfer to a pestle and mortar with the chilli and kaffir lime (add the ground turmeric now, if not using fresh) and pound to form a paste. Add the soy sauce and fish sauce (if using). Alternatively, blitz all the ingredients in a food processor.

Add the coconut cream at the end to round off the beautiful paste. Store in an airtight container in the fridge for up to 4 weeks.

Spices, dressings and pastes

Don't underestimate this classic, simple Asian dressing. Gingerols in ginger, vitamin C in lime and flavones in garlic are all potent, health-promoting ingredients and fantastic accompaniments to salads. I stir this through vegetables like chard, rocket and watercress or add it to brown rice noodles or simple steamed wholegrain rice. It is a fantastic, speedy dressing to have in your repertoire.

Asian Ginger and Soy Dressing

makes
about 75ml

50ml sesame oil (or melted coconut oil)

4cm piece of root ginger, peeled and grated

2 tsp honey

2 tbsp soy sauce

1 garlic clove, finely grated

juice of ½ lime

cayenne pepper or dried chilli flakes, to taste (optional)

Combine all the ingredients in a bowl and stir thoroughly. If you want to give the dressing a little heat, add a touch of cayenne or chilli flakes.

It will keep in an airtight container in the fridge for up to 1 week.

Spices, dressings and pastes

Tahini is full of essential fats and, combined with bitter greens such as kale, rocket and Brussels sprouts, actually aids the absorption of fat-soluble vitamins locked in their leaves. Vitamin C is richly concentrated in lemon juice and helps the absorption of iron found in greens, too. Stir this mix through your veggies and you can keep your friends guessing what the secret ingredients are.

makes about 50ml

Spiced Tahini Dressing

3 tbsp smooth tahini

2 tbsp cold-pressed sesame oil (or regular sesame oil)

1 tsp sumac

½ tsp cumin seeds, roughly ground

½ tsp dried chilli flakes

juice of ½ lemon, or to taste

Mix the tahini with the oil in a bowl until silky and smooth, then add the spices and chilli. Add lemon juice to taste (mixing the lemon juice into the dressing will thicken it).

It will keep in an airtight container in the fridge for up to 1 week.

Spices, dressings and pastes

In my family's house, we have a foodie game. Mum makes a chutney and my sister and I have to guess what she's put in it. The ingredient combinations are endless. A chutney is a fantastic way to get lots of fresh herbs into your diet. A combination of acidity, sweetness and fruit is all you need. Coriander and mint are some of the most common herbs available and are incredibly rich in antioxidants. Multiple scientific papers regard both these culinary herbs as potential 'nutraceuticals' – plants with potential use as medicine. Brimming with hundreds of phytochemicals, they are more powerful in combination than alone. Enjoy experimenting.

makes
about 300g

Medicinal Chutney

25g mint leaves

25g coriander leaves and stalks

1 tsp honey

1 green chilli, deseeded

50g pomegranate seeds
(or red seedless grapes)

150ml water

50g full-fat yoghurt (optional)

Put all the ingredients (except the yoghurt) in a blender or food processor and blitz to form a fine liquid. Add more water if needed.

Taste, and if you'd like the chutney to be milder, stir in the yoghurt.

The chutney will keep in the fridge for a few days, but try to make it fresh if possible.

TIP

+ I like to serve this as a dressing for my 'perfectly' cooked greens (see page 102) or as a delicious sauce for plain roasted sweet potato or grilled fish.

Spices, dressings and pastes

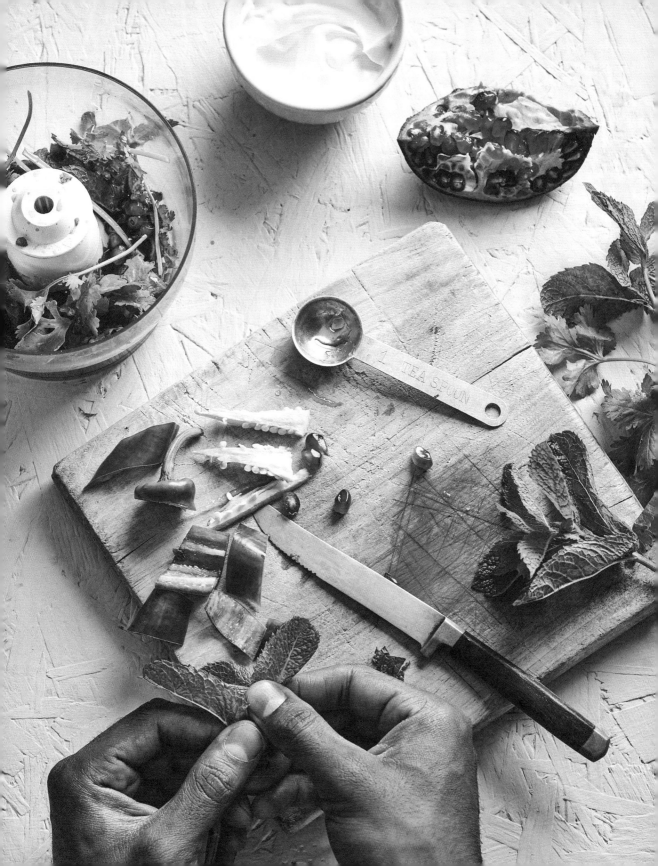

In my family home, oil flavoured with dried chilli and a little garlic has always been in our cupboards. Any simple steamed vegetables are transformed with oil blends. Best of all, blends of oil and spice made from scratch contain a variety of plant chemicals shown to offer health benefits, not to mention the polyphenols in good-quality extra-virgin olive oil itself. Meat, fish and vegetables all take well to oil blends, so do experiment!

Oil Blends

makes 200ml

200ml extra-virgin olive oil

2 tsp ground spice of your choice (see suggestions below)

Combine the oil and spice in a small glass bottle or a jar, then shake, seal and store in a cool, dark place. Shake again before using.

Garam Masala – a sweet aromatic blend that takes to dark greens very well (see page 240 for my own blend).

Harissa – smoky flavour with heat, lends itself to root vegetables or chicken (see page 245 for my own blend).

Za'atar – light and herby, perfect for cauliflower, chicory or steamed celeriac (see page 242 for my own blend).

Ras el Hanout – Middle Eastern-influenced garam masala is how I describe this spice mix. It works really well with chickpeas and quinoa.

Berbere – a punchy North African spice blend which is great for elevating white fish and sweet potatoes.

Togarashi – this Japanese 7-spice blend has a citrus edge and is perfect for dressing summer salads of fennel, cucumber and tomatoes.

Spices, dressings and pastes

If I know I need a good night's rest, I prepare well. I have an early meal, take a bath, put all electronic equipment away at least two hours before bed, read and make chamomile tea. It's been recognised for years that chamomile herbs may help induce sleep. GPs all over the country recommend it, as well as good 'sleep hygiene' practices. This is my twist on the common tea remedy that may help you get a good night's rest, too.

makes 1 cup

Night-time Tea

2 green cardamom pods

½ tsp fennel seeds

½ tsp loose-leaf chamomile tea or 1 chamomile teabag

1 tsp honey (optional)

Bruise the cardamom pods and fennel seeds in a pestle and mortar.

Put the camomile tea in a mug of hot water with the bruised spices and leave to steep for 5 minutes before drinking, adding honey if you wish.

TIP

+ Valerian root is also known to have a sedative effect and can be found in a few commercially available teas marketed for sleep. But if you have recurrent issues with sleep, speak to your doctor.

Spices, dressings and pastes

My idea of being healthy isn't to simply sling turmeric into everything! What I eat and drink has to be enjoyable and it's got to have a purpose beyond just medicine. It may sound a little strange, but this 'turmeric tonic', a family tradition, is a beautiful everyday drinking tea with ingredients that may calm the mind and general inflammation. Many believe it helps with migraines and this may have some grounding in the evidence. Ginger has been shown to be quite an effective anti-nausea agent, so it's reasonable to think migraine sufferers may find some benefits from drinking this blend. Feel free to add your own twist with dried rose petals or even black molasses.

makes about
50g spice blend

Haldi Tea

For the spice blend

4 tsp ground turmeric

4 tsp ground cinnamon

4 tsp ground star anise
   (or ground cloves)

1 tsp ground nutmeg

½ tsp ground black pepper

For the tea

1 thin slice of root ginger

1 tsp maple syrup

juice of ½ lime

Mix the spice blend ingredients together and keep them in an airtight jar for up to 6–8 weeks.

To make a mug of tea, add ½ teaspoon of the spice blend to a mug with the tea ingredients, add hot water and stir. Allow to brew for 2–3 minutes before drinking. Taste and add more sweetener if needed.

Spices, dressings and pastes

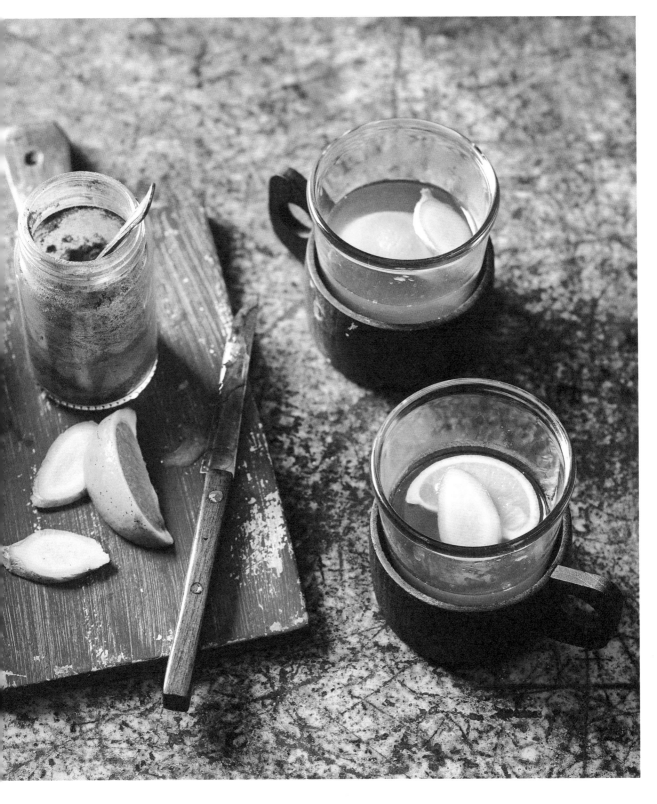

Spices, dressings and pastes

References

1. Karim SA, Ibrahim B, Tangiisuran B, Davies JG. What do healthcare providers know about nutrition support? A survey of the knowledge, attitudes and practice of pharmacists and doctors toward nutrition support in Malaysia. *J Parenter Enteral Nutr.* 2015;39(4):482–488.
2. Schwingshackl L, Hoffmann G. Adherence to Mediterranean diet and risk of cancer: a systematic review and meta-analysis of observational studies. *Int J Cancer.* 2014;135(8):1884–1897.
3. Esposito K, Maiorino M, Ciotola M, et al. Effects of a Mediterranean-style diet on the need for antihyperglycemic drug therapy in patients with newly diagnosed type 2 diabetes. *Ann Intern Med.* 2009;151(5):306.
4. Estruch R, Ros E, Salas-Salvadó J, et al. Primary prevention of cardiovascular disease with a Mediterranean diet. *N Engl J Med.* 2013;368(14):1279–1290.
5. Trichopoulou A, Costacou T, Bamia C, Trichopoulos D. Adherence to a Mediterranean diet and survival in a Greek population. *N Engl J Med.* 2003;348(26):2599.
6. Taylor R. Banting Memorial Lecture 2012: Reversing the twin cycles of type 2 diabetes. *Diabet Med.* 2013;30(3):267–275.
7. Knowler WC, Barrett-Connor E, Fowler SE, Hamman RF, Lachin JM, Walker EA NDDPPRG. Reduction in the incidence of type 2 diabetes with lifestyle intervention or metformin. *N Engl J Med.* 2006;346(6):393–403.
8. Bredesen DE. Reversal of cognitive decline: a novel therapeutic program. *Aging (Albany NY).* 2014;6(9):707–717.
9. Cai D, Feng W, Jiang Q. Acid-suppressive medications and risk of fracture: an updated meta-analysis. *Int J Clin Exp Med.* 2015;8(6):8893–8904.
10. Morgan L, Monica D. The economic burden of obesity. *Natl Obes Obs.* 2010;(October):1–13.
11. Diabetes UK. Facts and Stats. https://www.diabetes.org.uk/About_us/ What-we-say/Statistics/ Accessed: 13/07/2016.

12. Pathways NICE. Chronic heart failure overview. February 2016.
13. Pathways NICE. Population and community interventions. November 2016.
14. Pathways NICE. Cardiovascular disease prevention. June 2010.
15. Ray S, Laur C, Douglas P, et al. Nutrition education and leadership for improved clinical outcomes: training and supporting junior doctors to run 'Nutrition Awareness Weeks' in three NHS hospitals across England. *BMC Med Educ.* 2014;14(1):109.
16. Ray S, Udumyan R, Rajput-Ray M, et al. Evaluation of a novel nutrition education intervention for medical students from across England. *BMJ Open.* 2012;2:e000417.
17. Adams KM, Kohlmeier M, Zeisel SH. Nutrition education in US medical schools: latest update of a national survey. *Acad Med.* 2010;85(9): 1537–1542.
18. Kris-Etherton PM, Akabas SR, Douglas P, et al. Nutrition competencies in health professionals' education and training: a new paradigm. *Adv Nutr.* 2015;6:83–87.
19. British Heart Foundation. CVD Statistics – BHF UK Factsheet. 2016;(CVD).
20. Murakami A, Ohnishi K. Target molecules of food phytochemicals: food science bound for the next dimension. *Food Funct.* 2012;3(5):462.
21. Chen C. *Pigments in Fruits and Vegetables: Genomics and Dietetics*; 2015.
22. Cerella C, Sobolewski C, Dicato M, Diederich M. Targeting COX-2 expression by natural compounds: a promising alternative strategy to synthetic COX-2 inhibitors for cancer chemoprevention and therapy. *Biochem Pharmacol.* 2010;80(12):1801–1815.
23. Sacco SM, Horcajada M-N, Offord E. Phytonutrients for bone health during ageing. *Br J Clin Pharmacol.* 2013;75(3):697–707.

24. Thomas R, Williams M, Sharma H, Chaudry A, Bellamy P. A double-blind, placebo-controlled randomised trial evaluating the effect of a polyphenol-rich whole food supplement on PSA progression in men with prostate cancer – the UK NCRN Pomi-T study. *Prostate Cancer Prostatic Dis.* 2014;17(10): 180–186.
25. Dinu M, Abbate R, Gensini GF, Casini A, Sofi F. Vegetarian, vegan diets and multiple health outcomes: a systematic review with meta-analysis of observational studies. *Crit Rev Food Sci Nutr.* 2016;8398(February).
26. Health H, Hyson DA. A comprehensive review of apples and apple components and their relationship. 2011;1(3):408–420.
27. Liu RH. Dietary bioactive compounds and their health implications. *J Food Sci.* 2013;78(SUPPL.1).
28. Richter CK, Skulas-Ray AC, Champagne CM, Kris-Etherton PM. Plant protein and animal proteins: do they differentially affect cardiovascular disease risk? *Adv Nutr.* 2015;6(6): 712–728.
29. Oyebode O, Gordon-Dseagu V, Walker A, Mindell JS. Fruit and vegetable consumption and all-cause, cancer and CVD mortality: analysis of Health Survey for England data. *J Epidemiol Community Health.* 2014;68(9):856–862.
30. Tonstad S, Stewart K, Oda K, Batech M, Herring RP, Fraser GE. Vegetarian diets and incidence of diabetes in the Adventist Health Study-2. *Nutr Metab Cardiovasc Dis.* 2013;23(4):292–299.
31. Pereira PM de CC, Vicente AF dos RB. Meat nutritional composition and nutritive role in the human diet. *Meat Sci.* 2013;93(3):586–592.
32. Ruxton CHS, Derbyshire E, Pickard RS. Micronutrient challenges across the age spectrum: Is there a role for red meat? *Nutr Bull.* 2013;38(2):178–190.
33. Eaton SB. The ancestral human diet: what was it and should it be a paradigm for contemporary nutrition? *Proc Nutr Soc.* 2006;65(1):1–6.

34. Daley CA, Abbott A, Doyle PS, Nader GA, Larson S. A review of fatty acid profiles and antioxidant content in grass-fed and grain-fed beef. *Nutr J*. 2010;9:10.

35. Anand SS, Hawkes C, De Souza RJ, et al. Food consumption and its impact on cardiovascular disease: importance of solutions focused on the globalized food system. A report from the workshop convened by the World Heart Federation. *J Am Coll Cardiol*. 2015;66(14):1590–1614.

36. Davis C, Bryan J, Hodgson J, Murphy K. Definition of the Mediterranean diet: a literature review. *Nutrients*. 2015;7(11):9139–9153.

37. O'Hara AM, Shanahan F. The gut flora as a forgotten organ. *EMBO Rep*. 2006;7(7):688–693.

38. Vogt SL, Peña-Diaz J, Finlay BB. Chemical communication in the gut: effects of microbiota-generated metabolites on gastrointestinal bacterial pathogens. *Anaerobe*. 2015;34:106–115.

39. Ley R, Turnbaugh P, Klein S, Gordon J. Microbial ecology: human gut microbes associated with obesity. *Nature*. 2006;444(7122):1022–1023.

40. Round JL, Mazmanian SK. The gut microbiome shapes intestinal immune responses during health and disease. *Nat Rev Immunol*. 2009;9(5):313–323.

41. Mowat AM, Agace WW. Regional specialization within the intestinal immune system. *Nat Rev Immunol*. 2014;14(10):667–685.

42. Bhattacharjee S, Lukiw WJ. Alzheimer's disease and the microbiome. *Front Cell Neurosci*. 2013;7(September):153.

43. Davis CD. The gut microbiome and its role in obesity. *Nutr Today*. 2016;51(4):167–174.

44. Kitsios GD, Morowitz MJ, Dickson RP, Huffnagle GB, McVerry BJ, Morris A. Dysbiosis in the intensive care unit: microbiome science coming to the bedside. *J Crit Care*. 2016;38:84–91.

45. Graf D, Di Cagno R, Fåk F, et al. Contribution of diet to the composition of the human gut microbiota. *Microb Ecol Health Dis*. 2015;26:26164.

46. Slavin J. Fiber and prebiotics: mechanisms and health benefits. *Nutrients*. 2013;5(4):1417–1435.

47. Marelli G, Papaleo E, Ferrari A. Lactobacilli for prevention of urogenital infections: a review. *Eur Rev Med Pharmacol Sci*. 2004;8(2):87–95.

48. Aureli P, Capurso L, Castellazzi AM, et al. Probiotics and health: an evidence-based review. *Pharmacol Res*. 2011;63(5):366–376.

49. Johnson BC, Goldenberg JZ, Vandvik PO, Sun X, Guyatt GH. Probiotics for the prevention of pediatric antibiotic-associated diarrhea (Review). *Cochrane Database Syst Rev*. 2011;(11):1–49.

50. Hao Q, Dong BR, Wu T. Probiotics for preventing acute upper respiratory tract infections. *Cochrane Database Syst Rev*. 2015;(2):10–13.

51. Parvez S, Malik KA, Ah Kang S, Kim HY. Probiotics and their fermented food products are beneficial for health. *J Appl Microbiol*. 2006;100(6):1171–1185.

52. Chilton SN, Burton JP, Reid G. Inclusion of fermented foods in food guides around the world. *Nutrients*. 2015;7(1):390–404.

53. Veiga P, Pons N, Agrawal A, et al. Changes of the human gut microbiome induced by a fermented milk product. *Sci Rep*. 2014;4(6328):1–9.

54. Lee Y-K. Effects of diet on gut microbiota profile and the implications for health and disease. *Biosci microbiota, food Heal*. 2013;32(1):1–12.

55. Opara EI, Chohan M. Culinary herbs and spices: their bioactive properties, the contribution of polyphenols and the challenges in deducing their true health benefits. *Int J Mol Sci*. 2014;15(10):19183–19202.

56. Heiman ML, Greenway FL. A healthy gastrointestinal microbiome is dependent on dietary diversity. *Mol Metab*. 2016;5(5):317–320.

57. Glick-Bauer M, Yeh MC. The health advantage of a vegan diet: exploring the gut microbiota connection. *Nutrients*. 2014;6(11):4822–4838.

58. Matusheski N V, Juvik JA, Jeffery EH. Heating decreases epithiospecifier protein activity and increases sulforaphane formation in broccoli. *Phytochemistry*. 2004;65(9):1273–1281.

59. Hwang ES, Stacewicz-Sapuntzakis M, Bowen PE. Effects of heat treatment on the carotenoid and tocopherol composition of tomato. *J Food Sci*. 2012;77(10):1109–1114.

60. Jones RB, Frisina CL, Winkler S, Imsic M, Tomkins RB. Cooking method significantly effects glucosinolate content and sulforaphane production in broccoli florets. *Food Chem*. 2010;123(2):237–242.

61. Davies SC, Shallcross LJ. Antibiotic overuse. *Br J Gen Pract*. 2014;(December):604–605.

62. Francino MP. Antibiotics and the human gut microbiome: dysbioses and accumulation of resistances. *Front Microbiol*. 2016;6(JAN):1–11.

63. Frieri M, Kumar K, Boutin A. Antibiotic resistance. *J Infect Public Health*. 2017;10(4):369–378.

64. Ferrer M, Mendez-Garcia C, Rojo D, Barbas C, Moya A. Antibiotic use and microbiome function. *Biochem Pharmacol*. 2017;15(134):114–126.

65. Langdon A, Crook N, Dantas G. The effects of antibiotics on the microbiome throughout development and alternative approaches for therapeutic modulation. *Genome Med*. 2016;8(1):39.

66. Bengtsson-Palme J, Angelin M, Huss M, et al. The human gut microbiome as a transporter of antibiotic resistance genes between continents. *Antimicrob Agents Chemother*. 2015;59(10):6551–6560.

67. Jernberg C, Löfmark S, Edlund C, Jansson JK. Long-term impacts of antibiotic exposure on the human intestinal microbiota. *Microbiology*. 2010;156(11):3216–3223.

68. Suez J, Korem T, Zeevi D, et al. Artificial sweeteners induce glucose intolerance by altering the gut microbiota. *Nature*. 2014;514(7521):181–186.

69. Turnbaugh PJ, Ridaura VK, Faith JJ, Rey FE, Knight R, Gordon JI. The effect of diet on the human gut microbiome: a metagenomic analysis in humanized gnotobiotic mice. *Sci Transl Med*. 2009;1(6):6ra14.

70. Cerdá B, Pérez M, Pérez-Santiago JD, Tornero-Aguilera JF, González-Soltero R, Larrosa M. Gut microbiota modification: another piece in the puzzle of the benefits of physical exercise in health? *Front Physiol*. 2016;7(February):51.

71. Minich DM, Bland JS. Personalized lifestyle medicine: relevance for nutrition and lifestyle recommendations. *Sci World J*. 2013;2013.

72. Wahls TL. The seventy percent solution. *J Gen Intern Med*. 2011;26(10):1215–1216.

73. Ornish D, Magbanua MJM, Weidner G, et al. Changes in prostate gene expression in men undergoing an intensive nutrition and lifestyle intervention. *Proc Natl Acad Sci USA*. 2008;105(24):8369–8374.

74. Ornish D, Lin J, Chan JM, et al. Effect of comprehensive lifestyle changes on telomerase activity and telomere length in men with biopsy-proven low-risk prostate cancer: 5-year follow-up of a descriptive pilot study. *Lancet Oncol*. 2013;14(11):1112–1120.

75. Bohn SK, Myhrstad MC, Thoresen M, et al. Blood cell gene expression associated with cellular stress defense is modulated by antioxidant-rich food in a randomised controlled clinical trial of male smokers. *BMC Med*. 2010;8:54.

76. Ornish D. Mostly plants. *Am J Cardiol*. 2009;104(7):957–958.

77. Zeevi D, Korem T, Zmora N, et al. Personalized nutrition by prediction of glycemic responses. *Cell*. 2015;163(5):1079–1095.

78. Wong CP, Hsu A, Buchanan A, et al. Effects of sulforaphane and 3,3'-diindolylmethane on genome-wide promoter methylation in normal prostate epithelial cells and prostate cancer cells. *PLoS One*. 2014;9(1).

79. Arigony ALV, De Oliveira IM, Machado M, et al. The influence of micronutrients in cell culture: a reflection on viability and genomic stability. *Biomed Res Int*. 2013;2013.

80. Duthie SJ, Narayanan S, Brand GM, Pirie L, Grant G. Impact of folate deficiency on DNA stability. *J Nutr*. 2002;132:2444S–2449S.

81. Farzaei MH, Abbasabadi Z, Ardekani MRS, Rahimi R, Farzaei F. Parsley: a review of ethnopharmacology, phytochemistry and biological activities. *J Tradit Chinese Med*. 2013;33(6): 815–826.

82. Lin Y, Shi R, Wang X, Shen H-M. Luteolin, a flavonoid with potential for cancer prevention and therapy. *Curr Cancer Drug Targets*. 2008;8(7): 634–646.

83. Bumke-Vogt C, Osterhoff MA, Borchert A, et al. The flavones apigenin and luteolin induce FOXO1 translocation but inhibit gluconeogenic and lipogenic gene expression in human cells. *PLoS One*. 2014;9(8):e104321.

84. Ullah MF, Khan MW. Food as medicine: potential therapeutic tendencies of plant derived polyphenolic compounds. *Asian Pacific J Cancer Prev*. 2008;9(2):187–196.

85. Miller AH, Raison CL. The role of inflammation in depression: from evolutionary imperative to modern treatment target. *Nat Rev Immunol*. 2016;16(1):22–34.

86. Horbowicz M, Kosson R, Grzesiuk A, Dębski H. Anthocyanins of fruits and vegetables: their occurrence, analysis and role in human nutrition. *Veg Crop Res Bull*. 2008;68(1):5–22.

87. Wang L-S, Stoner GD. Anthocyanins and their role in cancer prevention. *Cancer Lett*. 2008;269(2):281–290.

88. Link A, Balaguer F, Goel A. Cancer chemoprevention by dietary polyphenols: promising role for epigenetics. *Biochem Pharmacol*. 2010;80(12):1771–1792.

89. Blekhman R, Goodrich JK, Huang K, et al. Host genetic variation impacts microbiome composition across human body sites. *Genome Biol*. 2015;16(1):191.

90. Krautkramer KA, Kreznar JH, Romano KA, et al. Diet-microbiota interactions mediate global epigenetic programming in multiple host tissues. *Mol Cell*. 2016;64(5):982–992.

91. Sonnenburg JL, Bäckhed F. Diet–microbiota interactions as moderators of human metabolism. *Nature*. 2016;535(7610):56–64.

92. Jeffery IB, O'Toole PW. Diet–microbiota interactions and their implications for healthy living. *Nutrients*. 2013;5(1):234–252.

93. Oike H, Oishi K, Kobori M. Nutrients, clock genes and chrononutrition. *Curr Nutr Rep*. 2014;3:204–212.

94. Korkmaz A, Rosales-Corral S, Reiter RJ. Gene regulation by melatonin linked to epigenetic phenomena. *Gene*. 2012;503(1):1–11.

95. Carpentieri A, Díaz De Barboza G, Areco V, Peralta López M, Tolosa De Talamoni N. New perspectives in melatonin uses. *Pharmacol Res*. 2012;65(4):437–444.

96. Hirschey MD, Shimazu T, Goetzman E, et al. SIRT3 regulates fatty acid oxidation via reversible enzyme deacetylation. 2010;464(7285): 121–125.

97. Wegman MP, Guo M, Bennion DM, et al. Practicality of intermittent fasting in humans and its effect on oxidative stress and genes related to aging and metabolism. *Rejuvenation Res*. 2014;18(352):1–50.

98. Wijngaarden MA, van der Zon GC, van Dijk KW, Pijl H, Guigas B. Effects of prolonged fasting on AMPK signaling, gene expression and mitochondrial respiratory chain content in skeletal muscle from lean and obese individuals. *Am J Physiol Endocrinol Metab*. 2013;304(9):E1012–21.

99. Martin B, Mattson MP, Maudsley S. Caloric restriction and intermittent fasting: two potential diets for successful brain aging. *Ageing Res Rev*. 2006;5(3):332–353.

100. Deng W, Cheung ST, Tsao SW, Wang XM, Tiwari AFY. Telomerase activity and its association with psychological stress, mental disorders, lifestyle factors and interventions: a systematic review. *Psychoneuroendocrinology*. 2015;64:150–163.

101. Rao KS, Chakrabarti SK, Dongare VS, et al. An intensive mind and body therapeutic program leads to alteration in gene expression critical to aging process in peripheral blood stem cells. *Adv Aging Res*. 2015;4(3):89–95.

102. Schutte NS, Malouff JM. A meta-analytic review of the effects of mindfulness meditation on telomerase activity. *Psychoneuroendocrinology*. 2014;42:45–48.

103. Jonsson T, Granfeldt Y, Ahren B, et al. Beneficial effects of a Paleolithic diet on cardiovascular risk factors in type 2 diabetes: a randomized cross-over pilot study. *Cardiovasc Diabetol*. 2009;8(1):35.

104. Masharani U, Sherchan P, Schloetter M, et al. Metabolic and physiologic effects from consuming a hunter-gatherer (Paleolithic)-type diet in type 2 diabetes. *Eur J Clin Nutr*. 2015;69(November 2014):1–5.

105. Bisht B, Darling WG, Grossmann RE, et al. A multimodal intervention for patients with secondary progressive multiple sclerosis: feasibility and effect on fatigue. *J Altern Complement Med*. 2014;20(5):347–355.

106. Masino SA, Ruskin DN. Ketogenic diets and pain. *J Child Neurol*. 2013;28(8):993–1001.

107. Barañano KW, Hartman AL. The ketogenic diet: uses in epilepsy and other neurologic illnesses. *Curr Treat Options Neurol*. 2008;10(6):410–419.

108. Paoli A, Rubini A, Volek JS, Grimaldi KA. Beyond weight loss: a review of the therapeutic uses of very-low-carbohydrate (ketogenic) diets. *Eur J Clin Nutr*. 2013;67(8):789–796.

109. Mavropoulos JC, Yancy WS, Hepburn J, Westman EC. The effects of a low-carbohydrate, ketogenic diet on the polycystic ovary syndrome: a pilot study. *Nutr Metab (Lond)*. 2005;2(1):1–5.

110. Gower BA, Chandler-Laney PC, Ovalle F, et al. Favourable metabolic effects of a eucaloric lower-carbohydrate diet in women with PCOS. *Clin Endocrinol (Oxf)*. 2013;79(4):550–557.

111. Gannon MC, Nuttall FQ. Amino acid ingestion and glucose metabolism: a review. *IUBMB Life*. 2010;62(9): 660–668.

112. Aune D, Chan DSM, Lau R, et al. Dietary fibre, whole grains and risk of colorectal cancer: systematic review and dose-response meta-analysis of prospective studies. *BMJ*. 2011;343:d6617.

113. Dang W. The controversial world of sirtuins. *Drug Discov Today Technol*. 2014;12:e9–e17.

114. Landecker H. Food as exposure: nutritional epigenetics and the new metabolism. *Biosocieties*. 2011;6(2):167–194.

115. Choi S-W, Friso S. Epigenetics: a new bridge between nutrition and health. *Adv Nutr*. 2010;1(1):8–16.

116. Mattson MP, Wan R. Beneficial effects of intermittent fasting and caloric restriction on the cardiovascular and cerebrovascular systems. *J Nutr Biochem*. 2005;16(3):129–137.

117. Harvie M, Wright C, Pegington M, et al. The effect of intermittent energy and carbohydrate restriction v. daily energy restriction on weight loss and metabolic disease risk markers in overweight women. *Br J Nutr*. 2013;110(8): 1534–1547.

118. Harvie MN, Sims AH, Pegington M, et al. Intermittent energy restriction induces changes in breast gene expression and systemic metabolism. *Breast Cancer Res*. 2016;18(1):57.

119. Johnstone A. Fasting for weight loss: an effective strategy or latest dieting trend? *Int J Obes*. 2015;39(5):727–733.

120. Mercken EM, Carboneau BA, Krzysik-Walker SM, De Cabo R. Of mice and men: the benefits of caloric restriction, exercise and mimetics. *Ageing Res Rev*. 2012;11(3): 390–398.

121. Longo VD, Panda S. Fasting, circadian rhythms, and time-restricted feeding in healthy lifespan. *Cell Metab*. 2016;23(6):1048–1059.

122. Rothschild J, Hoddy KK, Jambazian P, Varady KA. Time-restricted feeding and risk of metabolic disease: a review of human and animal studies. *Nutr Rev*. 2014;72(5):308–318.

123. Bonjour J-P. Nutritional disturbance in acid-base balance and osteoporosis: a hypothesis that disregards the essential homeostatic role of the kidney. *Br J Nutr*. 2013;110(7): 1168–1177.

124. Schwalfenberg GK. The alkaline diet: is there evidence that an alkaline pH diet benefits health? *J Environ Public Health*. 2012;2012.

125. Pizzorno J, Frassetto LA, Katzinger J. Diet-induced acidosis: is it real and clinically relevant? *Br J Nutr*. 2010;103(8):1185–1194.

126. Kellum JA. Determinants of blood pH in health and disease. *Crit Care*. 2000;4(1):6–14.

127. Remer T. Influence of diet on acid-base balance. *Semin Dial*. 2000;13(4):221–226.

128. Fenton TR, Huang T. Systematic review of the association between dietary acid load, alkaline water and cancer. *BMJ Open*. 2016;6(6):e010438.

129. Vormann J, Goedecke T. Latent acidosis: overacidification as a cause of chronic diseases. *Schweiz Zschr Ganzheitsmedizin*. 2002;14(January 2002):90–96.

130. Luke A, Cooper RS. Physical activity does not influence obesity risk: time to clarify the public health message. *Int J Epidemiol*. 2013;42(6):1831–1836.

131. Alpert W, Look AHEAD Research Group. Cardiovascular effects of intensive lifestyle intervention in Type 2 diabetes. *N Engl J Med*. 2013;369: 145–154.

132. Howard BV, Horn V, Hsia J, et al. Low-fat dietary pattern and risk of cardiovascular disease. *J Am Med Assoc*. 2006;295(6):655–666.

133. Delas I. Benefits and hazards of fat-free diets. *Trends Food Sci Technol*. 2011;22(10):576–582.

134. Atrens DM. The questionable wisdom of a low-fat reduction diet. *Soc Sci Med*. 1994;39(3):433–447.

135. Harcombe Z, Baker JS, Davies B. Food for thought: have we been giving the wrong dietary advice? *Food Nutr Sci*. 2013;4(March):240–244.

136. Siri-tarino PW, Sun Q, Hu FB, Krauss RM. Saturated fat, carbohydrate, and cardiovascular disease. *Am J Clin Nutr*. 2010;(5):502–509.

137. de Souza RJ, Mente A, Maroleanu A, et al. Intake of saturated and trans unsaturated fatty acids and risk of all cause mortality, cardiovascular disease, and type 2 diabetes: systematic review and meta-analysis of observational studies. *BMJ*. 2015;351:1–16.

138. Chan RSM, Woo J. Prevention of overweight and obesity: how effective is the current public health approach. *Int J Environ Res Public Health*. 2010;7(3):765–783.

139. Ornish D, Scherwitz LW, Billings JH, et al. Intensive lifestyle changes for reversal of coronary heart disease. *Jama*. 1998;280(23):2001–2007.

140. St-Onge MP, Zhang S, Darnell B, Allison DB. Baseline serum C-reactive protein is associated with lipid responses to low-fat and high-polyunsaturated fat diets. *J Nutr*. 2009;139(4):680–683.

141. Giugliano D, Ceriello A, Esposito K. The effects of diet on inflammation. emphasis on the metabolic syndrome. *J Am Coll Cardiol*. 2006;48(4): 677–685.

142. Ravnskov U, Diamond DM, Hama R, et al. Lack of an association or an inverse association between low-density-lipoprotein cholesterol and mortality in the elderly: a systematic review. *BMJ Open*. 2016;6(6):e010401.

143. Kristensen ML, Christensen PM, Hallas J. The effect of statins on average survival in randomised trials, an analysis of end point postponement: Table 1. *BMJ Open*. 2015;5(9):e007118.

144. Sachdeva A, Cannon CP, Deedwania PC, et al. Lipid levels in patients hospitalized with coronary artery disease: an analysis of 136,905 hospitalizations in Get With the Guidelines. *Am Heart J*. 2009;157(1):111–117.e2.

145. Tantamango-Bartley Y, Jaceldo-Siegl K, Fan J, Fraser G. Vegetarian diets and the incidence of cancer in a low-risk population. *Cancer Epidemiol Biomarkers Prev*. 2013;22(2):286–294.

146. Rizzo NS, Sabaté J, Jaceldo-Siegl K, Fraser GE. Vegetarian dietary patterns are associated with a lower risk of metabolic syndrome: The Adventist Health Study 2. *Diabetes Care*. 2011;34(5):1225–1227.

147. Huang T, Yang B, Zheng J, Li G, Wahlqvist ML, Li D. Cardiovascular disease mortality and cancer incidence in vegetarians: a meta-analysis and systematic review. *Ann Nutr Metab*. 2012;60(4):233–240.

148. Key TJ, Appleby PN, Rosell MS. Health effects of vegetarian and vegan diets. *Proc Nutr Soc*. 2006;65(1): 35–41.

149. Nuttall FQ. Body mass index. *Medlin Plus*. 2012;50(3).

150. Bacon L, Aphramor L. Weight science: evaluating the evidence for a paradigm shift. *Nutr J*. 2011;10(1):9.

151. Ghosh S, Banerjee S, Sil PC. The beneficial role of curcumin on inflammation, diabetes and neurodegenerative disease: a recent update. *Food Chem Toxicol*. 2015;83:111–124.

152. Nelson KM, Dahlin JL, Bisson J, Graham J, Pauli GF, Walters MA. The essential medicinal chemistry of curcumin. *J Med Chem*. 2017:acs. jmedchem.6b00975.

153. Gupta SC, Patchva S, Aggarwal BB. Therapeutic roles of curcumin: lessons learned from clinical trials. *AAPS J*. 2013;15(1):195–218.

154. Prasad S, Tyagi AK, Aggarwal BB. Recent developments in delivery, bioavailability, absorption and metabolism of curcumin: the golden pigment from golden spice. *Cancer Res Treat*. 2014;46(1):2–18.

155. Bayan L, Koulivand PH, Gorji A. Garlic: a review of potential therapeutic effects. *Avicenna J Phytomed*. 2014;4(1):1–14.

156. Bozin B, Mimica-Dukic N, Samojlik I, Goran A, Igic R. Phenolics as antioxidants in garlic (*Allium sativum* L., Alliaceae). *Food Chem*. 2008;111(4):925–929.

157. Ried K, Fakler P. Potential of garlic (*Allium sativum*) in lowering high blood pressure: Mechanisms of action and clinical relevance. *Integr Blood Press Control*. 2014;7:71–82.

158. Rivlin RS. Recent advances on the nutritional effects associated with the use of garlic as a supplement: historical perspective on the use of garlic. *J Nutr*. 2001;131(1985):951–954.

159. Kolida S, Tuohy K, Gibson GR. Prebiotic effects of inulin and oligofructose. *Br J Nutr*. 2002;87(S2):S193–S197.

160. Duda-Chodak A, Tarko T, Satora P, Sroka P. Interaction of dietary compounds, especially polyphenols, with the intestinal microbiota: a review. *Eur J Nutr*. 2015;54(3):325–341.

161. Yekta ZP, Ebrahimi SM, Hosseini M, et al. Ginger as a miracle against chemotherapy-induced vomiting. *Iran J Nurs Midwifery Res*. 2012;17(5): 325–329.

162. Kubra IR, Rao LJM. An impression on current developments in the technology, chemistry and biological activities of ginger (*Zingiber officinale* Roscoe). *Crit Rev Food Sci Nutr*. 2012;52(8):651–688.

163. Leiherer A, Mundlein A, Drexel H. Phytochemicals and their impact on adipose tissue inflammation and diabetes. *Vascul Pharmacol*. 2013;58 (1–2):3–20.

164. Chakraborty A, Ferk F, Simić T, et al. DNA-protective effects of sumach (*Rhus coriaria* L.), a common spice: results of human and animal studies. *Mutat Res – Fundam Mol Mech Mutagen*. 2009;661(1–2):10–17.

165. Kosar M, Bozan B, Temelli F, Baser KHC. Antioxidant activity and phenolic composition of sumac (*Rhus coriaria* L.) extracts. *Food Chem*. 2007;103(3): 952–959.

166. Shidfar F, Rahideh ST, Rajab A, et al. The effect of sumac (*Rhus coriaria* L.) powder on serum glycemic status, ApoB, ApoA-I and total antioxidant capacity in type 2 diabetic patients. *Iran J Pharm Res IJPR*. 2014;13(4):1249–1255.

167. Salimi Z, Eskandary A, Headari R, Nejati V, Moradi M, Kalhori Z. Antioxidant effect of aqueous extract of sumac (*Rhus coriaria* L.) in the alloxan-induced diabetic rats. 2015;59(1):87–93.

168. Rayne S, Mazza G. Biological activities of extracts from sumac (*Rhus* spp.): a review. *Plant Foods Hum Nutr*. 2007;62(4):165–175.

169. Mnif S, Aifa S. Cumin (*Cuminum cyminum* L.) from traditional uses to potential biomedical applications. *Chem Biodivers*. 2015;12(5):733–742.

170. Zare R, Heshmati F, Fallahzadeh H, Nadjarzadeh A. Effect of cumin powder on body composition and lipid profile in overweight and obese women. *Complement Ther Clin Pract*. 2014;20(4):297–301.

171. Gachkar L, Yadegari D, Rezaei MB, Taghizadeh M, Astaneh SA, Rasooli I.

Chemical and biological characteristics of *Cuminum cyminum* and *Rosmarinus officinalis* essential oils. *Food Chem*. 2007;102(3):898–904.

172. Thippeswamy NB, Naidu KA. Antioxidant potency of cumin varieties – cumin, black cumin and bitter cumin – on antioxidant systems. *Eur Food Res Technol*. 2005;220(5–6):472–476.

173. Jungbauer A, Medjakovic S. Anti-inflammatory properties of culinary herbs and spices that ameliorate the effects of metabolic syndrome. *Maturitas*. 2012;71(3):227–239.

174. Mata AT, Proença C, Ferreira AR, Serralheiro MLM, Nogueira JMF, Araújo MEM. Antioxidant and antiacetylcholinesterase activities of five plants used as Portuguese food spices. *Food Chem*. 2007;103(3):778–786.

175. Van Puyvelde K, Mets T, Njemini R, Beyer I, Bautmans I. Effect of advanced glycation end product intake on inflammation and aging: a systematic review. *Nutr Rev*. 2014;72(10): 638–650.

176. Dog TL. A reason to season: the therapeutic benefits of spices and culinary herbs. *Explor J Sci Heal*. 2006;2(5):446–449.

177. Srinivasan K. Antioxidant potential of spices and their active constituents. *Crit Rev Food Sci Nutr*. 2012;54(3): 352–372.

178. Callaway JC. Hempseed as a nutritional resource: an overview. *Euphytica*. 2004:65–72.

179. Rodriguez-Leyva D, Pierce GN. The cardiac and haemostatic effects of dietary hempseed. *Nutr Metab (Lond)*. 2010;7(1):32.

180. House JD, Neufeld J, Leson G. Evaluating the quality of protein from hemp seed (*Cannabis sativa, L.*) products through the use of the protein digestibility-corrected amino acid score method. *J Agric Food Chem*. 2010;58(22):11801–11807.

181. Lecumberri E, Mateos R, Izquierdo-Pulido M, Rupérez P, Goya L, Bravo L. Dietary fibre composition, antioxidant capacity and physico-chemical properties of a fibre-rich product from cocoa (*Theobroma cacao, L.*). *Food Chem*. 2007;104(3):948–954.

182. Corti R, Flammer AJ, Hollenberg NK, Luscher TF. Cocoa and cardiovascular health. *Circulation*. 2009;119(10):1433–1441.

References

183. Latif R. Health benefits of cocoa. *Curr Opin Clin Nutr Metab Care.* 2013;16(6):669–674.

184. Sudarma V, Sukmaniah S, Siregar P. Effect of dark chocolate on nitric oxide serum levels and blood pressure in prehypertension subjects. *Acta Med Indones.* 2011;43(4):224–228.

185. Nehlig A. The neuroprotective effects of cocoa flavanol and its influence on cognitive performance. *Br J Clin Pharmacol.* 2013;75(3):716–727.

186. Chenopodium Q, Graf BL, Rojas-Silva P, et al. Innovations in health value and functional food development of quinoa (*Chenopodium quinoa Willd.*). 2016;14(4):431–445.

187. Vega-Glvez A, Miranda M, Vergara J, Uribe E, Puente L, Martínez EA. Nutrition facts and functional potential of quinoa (*Chenopodium quinoa Willd.*), an ancient Andean grain: a review. *J Sci Food Agric.* 2010;90(15):2541–2547.

188. Simnadis TG, Tapsell LC, Beck EJ. Physiological effects associated with quinoa consumption and implications for research involving humans: a review. *Plant Foods Hum Nutr.* 2015;70(3):238–249.

189. Guasch-Ferré M, Hu FB, Martínez-González MA, et al. Olive oil intake and risk of cardiovascular disease and mortality in the PREDIMED Study. *BMC Med.* 2014;12:78.

190. Venturini D, Simão ANC, Urbano MR, Dichi I. Effects of extra virgin olive oil and fish oil on lipid profile and oxidative stress in patients with metabolic syndrome. *Nutrition.* 2015;31(6):834–840.

191. Oliveras-López MJ, Berná G, Jurado-Ruiz E, López-García de la Serrana H, Martín F. Consumption of extra-virgin olive oil rich in phenolic compounds has beneficial antioxidant effects in healthy human adults. *J Funct Foods.* 2014;10:475–484.

192. Santos CSP, Cruz R, Cunha SC, Casal S. Effect of cooking on olive oil quality attributes. *Food Res Int.* 2013;54(2):2016–2024.

193. Piroddi M, Albini A, Fabiani R, et al. Nutrigenomics of extra-virgin olive oil: a review. *BioFactors.* 2016;(June 2016):17–41.

194. Li WW, Li VW, Hutnik M, Chiou AS. Tumor angiogenesis as a target for dietary cancer prevention. *J Oncol.* 2012;2012.

195. Johnson JJ, Bailey HH, Mukhtar H. Green tea polyphenols for prostate cancer chemoprevention: a translational perspective. *Phytomedicine.* 2010;17(1):3–13.

196. Chacko SM, Thambi PT, Kuttan R, Nishigaki I. Beneficial effects of green tea: a literature review. *Chin Med.* 2010;5(13):1–9.

197. N, Khan MH. Multitargeted therapy of cancer by green tea. *Cancer Lett.* 2008;269(2):269–280.

198. Weiss DJ, Anderton CR. Determination of catechins in matcha green tea by micellar electrokinetic chromatography. *J Chromatogr A.* 2003;1011:173–180.

199. Rodriguez-Leyva D, Dupasquier CMC, McCullough R, Pierce GN. The cardiovascular effects of flaxseed and its omega-3 fatty acid, alpha-linolenic acid. *Can J Cardiol.* 2010;26(9):489–496.

200. Kajla P, Sharma A, Sood DR. Flaxseed – a potential functional food source. *J Food Sci Technol.* 2015;52(4):1857–1871.

201. Hutchins AM, Brown BD, Cunnane SC, Domitrovich SG, Adams ER, Bobowiec CE. Daily flaxseed consumption improves glycemic control in obese men and women with pre-diabetes: a randomized study. *Nutr Res.* 2013;33(5):367–375.

202. Basu A, Rhone M, Lyons TJ. Berries: emerging impact on cardiovascular health. *Nutr Rev.* 2010;68(3):168–177.

203. Subash S, Essa MM, Al-Adawi S, Memon MA, Manivasagam T, Akbar M. Neuroprotective effects of berry fruits on neurodegenerative diseases. *Neural Regen Res.* 2014;9(16):1557–1566.

204. Devore EE, Kang JH, Breteler MMB, Grodstein F. Dietary intake of berries and flavonoids in relation to cognitive decline. *Ann Neurol.* 2013;72(1):135–143.

205. Del Bo' C, Martini D, Porrini M, Klimis-Zacas D, Riso P. Berries and oxidative stress markers: an overview of human intervention studies. *Food Funct.* 2015;6(9):2890–2917.

206. Michalska A, Łysiak G. Bioactive compounds of blueberries: post-harvest factors influencing the nutritional value of products. *Int J Mol Sci.* 2015;16(8):18642–18663.

207. Zava TT, Zava DT. Assessment of Japanese iodine intake based on seaweed consumption in Japan: a literature-based analysis. *Thyroid Res.* 2011;4:14.

208. Rupérez P. Mineral content of edible marine seaweeds. *Food Chem.* 2002;79(1):23–26.

209. Luca F, Perry G, Di Rienzo A. *Evolutionary Adaptations to Dietary Changes.* 2010;30:291–314.

210. Crinnion WJ. Organic foods contain higher levels of certain nutrients, lower levels of pesticides, and may provide health benefits for the consumer. *Altern Med Rev.* 2010;15(1):4–12.

211. Barrett DM, Beaulieu JC, Shewfelt R. Color, flavor, texture and nutritional quality of fresh-cut fruits and vegetables: desirable levels, instrumental and sensory measurement, and the effects of processing. *Crit Rev Food Sci Nutr.* 2010;50(5):369–389.

212. Lee SK, Kader AA. Preharvest and postharvest factors influencing vitamin C content of horticultural crops. *Postharvest Biol Technol.* 2000;20(3):207–220.

213. Barański M, Średnicka-Tober D, Volakakis N, et al. Higher antioxidant and lower cadmium concentrations and lower incidence of pesticide residues in organically grown crops: a systematic literature review and meta-analyses. *Br J Nutr.* 2014;112(5):794–811.

214. Parrón T, Requena M, Hernándcz AF, Alarcón R. Environmental exposure to pesticides and cancer risk in multiple human organ systems. *Toxicol Lett.* 2014;230(2):157–165.

215. Engel LS, Hill DA, Hoppin JA, et al. Pesticide use and breast cancer risk among farmers' wives in the agricultural health study. *Am J Epidemiol.* 2005;161(2):121–135.

216. Jaga K, Dharmani C. The epidemiology of pesticide exposure and cancer: a review. *Rev Environ Health.* 2005;20(1):15–38.

217. Zahm SH, Ward MH. Pesticides and childhood cancer. In: *Environmental Health Perspectives.* Vol 106; 1998:893–908.

218. Macdiarmid JI. Seasonality and dietary requirements: will eating seasonal food contribute to health and environmental sustainability? *Proc Nutr Soc.* 2014;73(Nov. 2013):368–375.

219. Sapone A, Bai JC, Ciacci C, et al. Spectrum of gluten-related disorders: consensus on new nomenclature and classification. *BMC Med.* 2012;10(1):13.

220. Czaja-Bulsa G. Non coeliac gluten sensitivity – a new disease with gluten intolerance. *Clin Nutr*. 2015;34(2): 189–194.

221. Biesiekierski JR, Newnham ED, Irving PM, et al. Gluten causes gastrointestinal symptoms in subjects without celiac disease: a double-blind randomized placebo-controlled trial. *Am J Gastroenterol*. 2011;106(March 2010):1–7.

222. Vazquez-Roque M, Oxentenko AS. Nonceliac gluten sensitivity. *Mayo Clin Proc*. 2015;90(9):1272–1277.

223. Fasano A. Zonulin, regulation of tight junctions, and autoimmune diseases. *Ann N Y Acad Sci*. 2012;1258(1):25–33.

224. Bressan P, Kramer P. Bread and Other Edible Agents of Mental Disease. *Front Hum Neurosci*. 2016;10(March):130.

225. Daulatzai MA. Non-celiac gluten sensitivity triggers gut dysbiosis, neuroinflammation, gut-brain axis dysfunction and vulnerability for dementia. *CNS Neurol Disord Drug Targets*. 2015;14(1):110–131.

226. Nylund L, Kaukinen K, Lindfors K. The microbiota as a component of the celiac disease and non-celiac gluten sensitivity. *Clin Nutr Exp*. 2016;6: 17–24.

227. Clarys P, Deliens T, Huybrechts I, et al. Comparison of nutritional quality of the vegan, vegetarian, semi-vegetarian, pesco-vegetarian and omnivorous diet. *Nutrients*. 2014;6(3):1318–1332.

228. Muita JW. Micronutrients in health and disease. *East Afr Med J*. 2001;78(9):449–450.

229. Patel KR, Sobczyńska-Malefora A. The adverse effects of an excessive folic acid intake. *Eur J Clin Nutr*. 2016;(August):1–5.

230. Hubner RA, Houlston RS. Folate and colorectal cancer prevention. *Br J Cancer*. 2009;100(2):233–239.

231. Samani NJ, Tomaszewski M, Schunkert H. The personal genome –

the future of personalised medicine? *Lancet*. 2010;375(9725):1497–1498.

232. Kitsios GD, Kent DM. Personalised medicine: not just in our genes. *BMJ*. 2012;344:e2161–e2161.

233. Wu QJ, Xiang YB, Yang G, et al. Vitamin E intake and the lung cancer risk among female nonsmokers: a report from the Shanghai Women's Health Study. *Int J Cancer*. 2015;136(3): 610–617.

234. Huang H-YY, Caballero B, Chang S, et al. The efficacy and safety of multivitamin and mineral supplement use to prevent cancer and chronic disease in adults: a systematic review for a National Institutes of Health state-of-the-science conference. *Ann Intern Med*. 2006;145(5):372–385.

235. Woodside JV, McCall D, McGartland C, Young IS. Micronutrients: dietary intake v. supplement use. *Proc Nutr Soc*. 2005;64(4):543–553.

236. Hodges RE, Minich DM. Modulation of metabolic detoxification pathways using foods and food-derived components: a scientific review with clinical application. *J Nutr Metab*. 2015;2015.

237. Gambini J, Inglés M, Olaso G, et al. Properties of resveratrol: in vitro and in vivo studies about metabolism, bioavailability, and biological effects in animal models and humans. *Oxid Med Cell Longev*. 2015;2015:837042.

238. Luxwolda MF, Kuipers RS, Kema IP, Dijck-Brouwer DA, Muskiet FA. Traditionally living populations in East Africa have a mean serum 25-hydroxyvitamin D concentration of 115 nmol/l. *Br J Nutr*. 2012;108(9):1557–1561.

239. Bjelakovic G, Gludd LL, Nikolova D, et al. Vitamin D supplementation for prevention of mortality in adults (Review). 2014;(1).

240. Durup D, Jørgensen HL, Christensen J, Schwarz P, Heegaard AM, Lind B. A reverse J-shaped association of all-cause mortality with serum

25-hydroxyvitamin D in general practice: The CopD study. *J Clin Endocrinol Metab*. 2012;97(8):2644–2652.

241. Grant WB. An estimate of the global reduction in mortality rates through doubling vitamin D levels. *Eur J Clin Nutr*. 2011;65(9):1016–1026.

242. Woo KS, Kwok TCY, Celermajer DS. Vegan diet, subnormal vitamin B-12 status and cardiovascular health. *Nutrients*. 2014;6(8):3259–3273.

243. Dyall SC. Long-chain omega-3 fatty acids and the brain: a review of the independent and shared effects of EPA, DPA and DHA. *Front Aging Neurosci*. 2015;7(APR):1–15.

244. Cottin SC, Alsaleh A, Sanders TAB, Hall WL. Lack of effect of supplementation with EPA or DHA on platelet-monocyte aggregates and vascular function in healthy men. 1–3. *Nutr Metab Cardiovasc Dis*. 2016;26(8):1–9.

245. Sanders TA. Plant compared with marine n-3 fatty acid effects on cardiovascular risk factors and outcomes: what is the verdict? *Am J Clin Nutr*. 2014;3(100):453S–8S.

246. Freeman MP, Davis M, Sinha P, Wisner KL, Hibbeln JR, Gelenberg AJ. Omega-3 fatty acids and supportive psychotherapy for perinatal depression: a randomized placebo-controlled study. *J Affect Disord*. 2008;110(1–2): 142–148.

247. Bauer I, Hughes M, Rowsell R, et al. Omega-3 supplementation improves cognition and modifies brain activation in young adults. *Hum Psychopharmacol*. 2014;29(2):133–144.

248. Pu H, Guo Y, Zhang W, et al. Omega-3 polyunsaturated fatty acid supplementation improves neurologic recovery and attenuates white matter injury after experimental traumatic brain injury. *J Cereb Blood Flow Metab*. 2013;33(9):1474–1484.

249. Allen LH. How common is vitamin B-12 deficiency? *Am J Clin Nutr*. 2009;89(2):693S–6S.

Index

Acknowledgements

I have to start by thanking my gorgeous family. My baby sister Jasmin, my father Surinder and Mother Indy. I would be nothing without you all as a source of strength and support throughout my life. I owe everything to my upbringing, your words of wisdom, your guidance and tolerance. I love you all more than you can imagine and I treasure every moment we're together.

To my team at HarperCollins Thorsons, what a wonderful and exciting bunch of souls. You have helped me create something I'm truly proud of. It's been an absolute pleasure working with you all, especially under the direction of my publisher, Carolyn, who really saw the potential of *The Doctor's Kitchen* as an exciting and relevant book. The photographers, stylists, editors, cooks, strategy and sales team have all made me feel very welcome and I've loved working with you all.

To my agent, Becca Barr, who ambushed me on my return from Australia back in 2016! Your insight and expertise have been invaluable and it's been brilliant working with you this far. It's great being part of the team and I look forward to future projects.

To Carly Cook, my literary agent, who has been an immense source of guidance and support throughout this huge process. You really gave me the initial confidence I needed to convince me that I could write a book. I can't thank you enough for your direction, as well as friendship.

To Alice Liveing who first spotted me thousands of miles away while I was living in Australia. Little did I know, she had been prompting Carly Cook to contact me on my return! She was one of the first people to recognise the potential of *The Doctor's Kitchen* and totally understood my message from the start. I can't repay you enough.

To Dr Rangan Chatterjee, who I look up to as a medical colleague and fellow lifestyle medicine doctor. Your support and motivation have encouraged me to be more open and continue with my aspirations. I'm forever grateful for your brotherly advice and close friendship.

To Dr Hazel Wallace, 'The Food Medic', I'm inspired by you. I can't tell you how valuable it is to have as support another doctor who understands this crazy double life and I'm so glad you were one of the people on my leaving boat party in Sydney! Your friendship, advice and support are invaluable. I cherish them very much.

As a medical doctor, getting in front of a camera and putting myself on social media was a very exposing and vulnerable position to put myself in. Had it not been for the encouragement of a few friends to whom I sheepishly introduced *The Doctor's Kitchen* early on, I would never have done it. Thank you, Pat, Romy, Ollie, Lizzie, Fiona, Summy and Dylan for being positive souls. You pushed me to follow my passion.

I'm merely a reflection of all my past experiences: positive, negative and neutral. For every one of those experiences I'm grateful because it has brought me to this point and will continue to shape my future whatever that entails going forward. To the first few followers on social media, to the many after that, I am indebted to you. You have helped gather support for this important message that I hope to bring to the world and all the thank yous I could muster will never be enough.

The tireless efforts of researchers worldwide who have shaped our understanding of nutrition in medicine is one of the most important acknowledgements to make. Without the passion of these scientists we would have no insight into the power of food as medicine. Thank you for your continual hard work and I'll persevere in making it accessible and relevant to as many people as possible.